THE FINAL ACT OF LIVING
Reflections of a Long-Time Hospice Nurse

by
BARBARA KARNES, RN

Published and distributed by
Barbara Karnes Books, Inc.
PO Box 189
Depoe Bay, OR 97341

In some of my other written work I have received
letters questioning my correct use of pronouns. I
am stating for all those people who will be reading
this book and checking my grammar that I have
intentionally chosen to use the word "their" when a
singular he, she, him or her should be used. I think
there is nothing so distracting to the message being
conveyed as the author trying to be politically correct and using he/she or her/him.

Index

INTRODUCTION

NOTES:

In the late 1970's, the hospice concept was creeping its way across the United States. I had graduated from nursing school in 1962, walked away with my diploma and thought, "That's it, I made a huge mistake. Nursing was not what I thought it was going to be, I'm out of here. No more nursing for me."

Years later, I realized I could have been a social worker and been fulfilled. Instead I married, had children, and dabbled in interior decorating. Nursing did not re-enter my mind until I learned of hospice.

The hospice concept was everything I thought nursing was going to be. It was holistic. It involved all parts of a person--not just the physical, but emotional, mental, and even spiritual. It included the family and significant others. It avoided medical procedures whenever possible. It dealt in comfort and quality and, most of all, personhood. The hospice concept focused on people who happened to have a disease, not on a disease that a person had.

In 1980, I took a refresher course in nursing and headed for the nearest hospice. I started as a volunteer in a small hospice (all hospices were small then) and four months later I joined the staff as a part-time nurse of a two-person RN team. From then until 1994, I was a part of a hospice team either as a staff nurse, a clinical director or (for the last six years) as an executive director. Hospice was my avocation. I had found my purpose.

In the early 80's there wasn't Medicare certification. Reimbursement came from community donations, fundraising and memorials. There were no rules or regulations to follow; in fact, we generally made up protocol as we went along.

I would stand on each porch before knocking and say to myself, "Dear God, I seek to heal, not hurt."

Inside was strictly a "fly by the seat of your pants" operation. We used Bag Balm for skin care, mayonnaise jars for urinals, Brompton's for pain management, and bed pads hand-made from newspapers covered in old sheets. What we lacked in supplies and knowledge, we made up for with time and nurturing. We filled a gap left open by the medical community. We were not part of the medical community, we were outside of it.

I think one of the reasons I was so creative in the hospice environment was because I had never really been a part of the medical model. I brought with me few preconceived ideas and little conditioning of how to actually be a nurse when I began working in hospice.

When I was taking the nursing refresher course, I worked on the oncology floor. At report one morning there was talk of a gentleman who had expressed suicidal intentions. Of course a psychiatric work up had been ordered, and we were told to be watchful of the man in room ----. Later that afternoon I was walking down the hall when the man in room --- called to me and asked if I could talk to him for a moment. He sat on his bed, the tray table between us, and I sat in a chair.

He told me how his wife had died of cancer several years earlier. How his children were scattered around the country, busy with their lives and families. How he had been the sole caregiver of his wife and how hard it had been. He reminisced about his life, the good and the difficult times. He expressed his feeling about not putting his children through caring for him, now that he had cancer, the way he had cared for his wife.

There weren't any answers to give this man; he just needed a listener. When he was finished he thanked me for my time. As I stood to go, my instinct was to give him a hug and just hold him a bit, but the tray table was between us so I walked out of the room.

As I cried in the utility room, I realized I had let the tray table, which represented all the lectures about distancing and non-emotional involvement, come between me and another human being. I vowed I would not let that happen again. I would relate to people as people first, Barbara to person, and nurse to person second. Barbara as a person and Barbara as a nurse didn't have to be separate. I could do and be both. I vowed to be real, open, sincere, to play no games and tell no lies. I reasoned that if I could bring those qualities to my work, I couldn't go wrong. It may not be the way others approached nursing, but that didn't matter. I was going to forge new territory.

The first Thanksgiving after I started working for

hospice, I went home to visit my parents. I called back to check on some patients, and then shared with my mother that a particular patient had died. Her response was concern. "Are you sure you are doing everything right? All your patients are dying." Her reaction was so typical of how most people relate to death from disease. Doctors and nurses must be doing something wrong if the end result is death. I hoped to break that stereotype.

This book is a compilation of what I have learned throughout my years of working with people who were approaching death. All of my patients have died. They and their families have taught me more about living than any books or workshops I attended.

During the early years, before hourly wage regulations and workman's compensation were a part of hospice, whenever death was approaching, we simply stayed at the home for as long as necessary. I can't count the number of nights I slept on the floor beside a hospital bed in someone's bedroom or on a living room sofa. Families were not left alone with their fears. We couldn't take this difficult experience away, but we could be there and nurture. That was often the most we could offer. Comfort management still had a long way to grow.

I see hospice and palliative care today, twenty-three years later, and marvel at the medical changes. Today there is no reason for anyone to die in pain. We administer various forms of morphine in milligrams in the hundreds. (The first time I titrated a morphine level up to eighty milligrams, I was very concerned that my patient might die before my eyes of an overdose I had given him. He didn't; in fact, he got out of bed and moved around the house, comfortable for the first time in a long while.) We have special beds, endless skin care products, and every kind of nutritional supplement imaginable. All of this is directed toward comfort management.

We have Medicare, Medicaid and insurance reimbursement. There are Hospice Houses all over the country, as well as hospice in nursing facilities. The services we now provide are comprehensive. Hospice has become a part of the medical model. It is not outside of it any longer. It has gradually become more and more medically oriented.

From some standpoints, that is a positive advancement-- but there is a downside. In becoming part of the medical establishment, it is becoming harder and harder to concentrate on the person that has the disease as opposed to the disease that the person has.

With regulations come safeguards against fraud and abuse, but also a long list of protocols and policies, of forms and accountabilities that detract from the humanity and common sense that once was our main focus. Now fear of not meeting certain criteria keeps us from admitting patients instead of admitting on instinct and utilizing the Medicare 90 day recertification process for dismissing a person if they are no longer appropriate.

I talked to a gentleman in California who was starting a volunteer program to assist families of loved ones with a limited prognosis. I suggested hospice, to which he answered they had not met his need for succor, for compassion, for nurturing. Yes, they paid for the medications, they gave his wife a bath, they talked with his physician. But he wanted more.

Have we come full circle? Are we now so much a part of the medical model that we have obscured our original intent? Will people be forming programs under a different name than hospice to provide what we are now lacking? I don't have answers to those questions, but those questions are the reason I am writing this book. I don't want the simple way of viewing death, of caring for those at the end of their life, to get lost.

Growth and advancement are good. I am so glad we now have all of the resources that we offer to patients and families. I just don't want to lose our original intent of nurturing, of quality, of common sense, of open caring and support.

What follows in this book are the ideas, insights and experiences that I have gathered over these last twenty-three years. I do not pretend that what I am going to relate is the Truth with that capital "T". These are only my perceptions, my truths. You may disagree with some of my thoughts. My intent is to give you a different perspective, maybe a broader look, at living and at end of life issues. If you finish this book and say to yourself, "I hadn't thought about living and death that way before," then my purpose for writing will have been fulfilled.

DYNAMICS OF
APPROACHING DEATH

NOTES:

We don't have accurate role models on what it is to die. All we have is television, movies and any deathbed experience in which we have been involved.

If we have been at the bedside when someone was dying, we brought our own preconceived ideas, our fears, our culture, all of our life experiences with us. These beliefs influenced and distorted our perception of what was actually occurring. Now we will bring the memory of this distortion (only for us it will appear as actual) to any deathbed experience in the future, whether it be our own death, or the death of someone we care about. If our aunt Bertha died a painful death from cancer of the bone, we will expect to die a painful death even though we have cancer of the pancreas and it is fifteen years later. In fifteen years, pain management has drastically changed. There is no reason for someone to die in pain today.

And people don't die like they do on television or in the movies. There are two stereotypes that we associate with dying that we get from movies. Visualize a young Clint Eastwood; mom is dying, her sons, including Clint, are gathered around the bed. She is telling them something very profound; they are hanging on her every word. She comes to the end of her message, the end of her sentence, then--only then--she takes a deep breath, closes her mouth and eyes, drops her head to the side, and she is dead.

People don't die like that. They may be talking, but if they are, you probably can't hear them because they don't have enough energy to project their voice. If you can hear them, they probably aren't making any sense. They are so otherworldly that they are talking about the other world, not this one.

The other thing we expect to see at the bedside is this scenario, which comes from the movie

"Dangerous Liaisons." Michelle Pfiffer is dying; she is lying in her convent bed, looking magnificent - make up and hair perfect. (People who are dying don't look magnificent, in fact they don't look good at all. They look pale and gaunt. There may be a spiritual radiance about the person, but physically they don't look very good.) Anyway, the next scene shows Michelle with her eyes wide open in a blank stare. That is our message that she is dead. Now a hand passes across her face and her eyelids magically close and stay shut. In real life, yes, a person dies with their eyes open. Not wide-open, but with the eyelids partially open, kind of at half-mast. If you pass your hand in front of their eyes, of course nothing happens, and if you take your thumb and forefinger and close their eyelids, those eyelids are going to open right up again. That is when I have to scrape everyone off the ceiling because their role models tell them the eyes stay shut.

We used to have role models because grandma lived at home. We were multi-generational. When grandma got sick, she didn't go to the hospital, she went into the upstairs bedroom and there she died. When she died we didn't call a funeral home--instead we washed her body, dressed her in her Sunday dress, and laid her body out in the parlor or the living room. Family, friends, and neighbors came to the house to pay their respects. We learned how to die, and we learned how to grieve, because we were there.

Today, Grandma lives in a senior citizen high rise. When she gets sick she goes to a hospital, and from there to a nursing home. If she is lucky we visit her on Sundays after church, but more than likely we visit her on Thanksgiving, Christmas, Easter and Mother's Day. Then one day she is dead, and the next time we see her is in a coffin, in a funeral home, with a dress that we had to go out and buy for the occasion, with a hairdo that isn't grandma's and she probably has on too much makeup. We didn't learn how to die and we didn't learn how to grieve. Because of this lack of experience we approach one of the most normal, natural experiences of our lives totally unprepared.

Everyone dies! Dying is normal. It is natural. That is the one thing I can guarantee about this world. Everyone dies. Well, everybody except me. I'm not going to die and neither is anyone close to me. Other people die.

If I were to be diagnosed with a life threatening illness, the doctors would be wrong. If I were diagnosed with a life threatening illness, there would be a cure discovered before I died. If both of those fail, then there will be a miracle. God is not going to let me die.

I don't think I am any different for anyone else. We cannot comprehend our own death. Other people die. We can be told, "You have a life threatening illness. Go home, put your affairs in order." I can prepare my will, write my obituary, and tell you that I can't be fixed but that doesn't mean I believe it. I have it in my head, mentally I know and hear all that is being said, but it is not in my heart. We cannot comprehend our own death!

There are just two ways to die--gradually and fast. It is so simple. Fast death is getting hit by a truck. It is a heart attack. It is suicide. You are alive one minute and dead the next. Fast death is harder on the survivors than it is on the person who died. We, the survivors, have a lot of unfinished business, a lot of guilt. And a lot of questions that have no answers. "What if?" "Why didn't I?" "If only." Those questions and the ensuing guilt will complicate our grieving and make it more difficult.

Gradual death comes in two ways, disease and old age. In old age our body simply wears out and dies.

The other way of gradual death is through disease. Disease is one of the ways the spirit chooses to get out of this body. One of the things I want you to remember is that this body is not who we are. I may think my body is Barbara Karnes. Well, my body is no more Barbara Karnes than my car is Barbara Karnes. My body is just a vehicle that Barbara Karnes uses to get around in on this planet. I can get out of this body just as easily as I can get out of my car; it is just that no one tells me how.

The only difference between death from old age and death from disease is time. A person who is just old with no disease process will take longer to die. Where a person with a disease will have certain signs for months, someone who is just old will have the same signs for years. A person who is old will have the signs of approaching death that signify weeks, last for months. When it gets down to days, hours and minutes we all die the same, including fast death.

I saw a television show where a camera crew accompanied paramedics for an evening. The paramedics were loading a guy into an ambulance to take him to the hospital. From the signs I saw, I knew he would probably not live to make it to the hospital. A different documentary showed a bird sitting on a rock with a plastic six-pack ring around its neck. By what the bird was doing sitting on that rock I knew the bird was dying. When it gets to days, hours and minutes, all of God's creatures die the same way.

There are very few Dying 101 classes that tell us what it is like to die. In fact, few people are comfortable enough to tell us we are going to die.

Imagine this scene: Mom is dying. She is in the bedroom; all the family is present, going in and out of the room. Outside mom's room everyone is crying, but when it is our turn to go into the bedroom we stop crying, stand up straight and walk to her bedside with a smile on our face. "Hey, Mom. How are you doing? You know if you will just eat you'll feel better. Why, we'll be in that shopping mall before you know it." You squeeze her hand, kiss her, tell her how much you love her. She smiles, playing this game with you, and then you leave the room and resume crying.

Nobody tells us when we are dying. Few people can say, "Mom, you're dying. I don't know when, but I know it's going to happen. Let's talk."

Gradual death gives us an opportunity to do and say those things we need to do and say, if we will take it. Most of us don't.

From this point forward, I am going to talk about dying from disease. As I said, there isn't a lot to discuss about fast death. You are alive then you are dead. Gradual death from old age or disease has a process to it. If it were happenstance, it would be fast death.

Dying a gradual death is a lot like infant development. Most babies roll over give or take a few weeks; most babies walk, give or take a few months. You always have the 9 month-old sitting on the floor who suddenly jumps up and runs across the room. You say, "He can't do that! He has to creep, and crawl and toddle first." Well, he didn't play by the rules.

You always have the person dying from disease or old age who is alive one minute and dead the next, who didn't play by the rules, but most people dying from disease or old age will do certain things at certain times.

We don't even have to know a person's diagnosis to tell if they have entered the dying process. We don't have to know their lab values. All we have to do is ask questions concerning three pertinent areas-- food, sleep and social interaction. Based on the responses we can pretty well tell if a person has months, weeks, days or hours to live.

Beware of anyone who puts a number on how long someone has to live. Each person dies in their own unique manner. That manner will fit within the time frame--but the dynamics of a person's life determine that time frame, not lab values or diagnosis.

When we put a number on how long someone has to live, we are doing that person a disservice. Because we don't have role models on what it is like to die, we think we are going to be alive one minute and dead the next. We don't know there is a process. Imagine the fear of waking up every morning and wondering if you are going to die that day. When I think that is happening, I tell a person with a life threatening illness, "If you can ask yourself 'Am I going to die today?' then you are probably not. The day that you die, you won't ask and you won't care." Think of the fear that this simple statement reduces.

An individual will die in their own unique way and in their own time. They will probably do certain things within a certain timeline, but it will hold to their personality and the individual way they have lived their life.

We die the same way that we have lived. Dying is just one more experience in this game called life. We will deal with it in the same way that we address all the other challenges of our life.

There are few deathbed conversions. You don't generally go from being ornery and cantankerous to being a saint. What usually happens is you go from being ornery and cantankerous to being an absolute monster. Dying doesn't change us; it intensifies our personality.

A Type A, doer personality will orchestrate their end of life. They will have their Living Will in place, their Durable Power of Attorney; they will pick out their cemetery plot, and may even write their obituary. The Type A personality, if they don't die of a heart attack, will probably develop a disease and die quickly. It would be absolutely intolerable for a Type A personality to be in bed for three months.

Someone who is more laid back, a little easier going, content to watch the soaps all afternoon, will develop a disease and die more slowly. There isn't a lot of difference sitting in your favorite recliner or being in bed.

We all know people who use manipulation to get what they want from life. People can use manipulation in their dying as well. How about the Mom who is dying; all of her kids are with her. "We'll stay with you as long as you need us," they tell her. Mom is not going to die quickly. She is probably getting more attention from her children in this dying process than she ever got through normal living.

Some people feel that if they talk about death and dying, then they will surely die. They are "going to beat this thing" throughout the entire course of the disease. That may be the attitude of a person who has denied other challenges in their life.

We have partial control over the time that we die. If there is something we need to do or say that is very important, we will try to stay here to complete our work. We've all heard the story of Dad being on death's door. The son is coming in from out of town, finally arrives, walks in, and says, "Dad I'm here," fifteen minutes later, Dad dies. He waited for his son to be there.

Or how about waiting by my Mom's bedside for days and leaving the room for a second only to return to find she has died. Oh, the guilt that goes with that occurrence. It is very important to know, if we are with someone when they die it is because they want us with them. If we are not with someone when they die they choose that also. We can take the gift of love and protection that they have given us. Protective parents tend to not die with their children in the room, even if that child is seventy years old.

Everyone, to some degree, is going to be afraid when it comes time to die. I am a nervous public speaker; it is what I do for a living, but every time I begin a presentation I am frightened. If I am frightened speaking in front of an audience, and I know the outcome will be fine, how will I feel when it comes time to die? I don't remember doing that before. Anytime we do something new, we are at least nervous--if not downright terrified.

I'll often hear when a person is talking about end of life issues that they are not afraid to die. As death becomes more of a reality, that same person becomes nervous and scared. Their first thought is that they are not strong enough in their religious beliefs, not close enough to their God, because if they were, they wouldn't be frightened now. The truth is, their fear has nothing to do with God. They are simply a human being facing the unknown. Everyone is going to be frightened as they approach gradual death. It will be just a question of degree.

Most of us are more afraid of the process of dying

than of being dead. My belief systems tell me that when I am dead, I will be in a better place. I am not really afraid of being dead. I am, however, afraid of the unknown space between now and the time I am dead.

I have often thought if God would say to me, "Barbara, you are going to die, and this is when you're going to die and how you're going to die," then I would relax, ride more roller coasters, live a freer life.

When a physician says, "Go home, put your affairs in order," isn't he really saying, "You're going to die, this is when and this is how?" Unfortunately, most people upon hearing this news go home, sit in their favorite recliner and might as well die that moment because they stop living and just wait to die. Their entire life becomes centered around the disease and dying. They waste precious, valuable time by not living until they are dead.

There is really no such action as dying. It is a misnomer. We use it to make reference to a process and a time period, but really there is no such thing. We are either alive or dead. The space in between is called living.

Life is a terminal illness. We are "dying" all the time. We are born, we experience, and then we die. The only difference between someone in a healthy body and someone in an unhealthy body is the person in the unhealthy body is reminded every day they are not going to live forever. We, on the other hand, live under the illusion that we, because we are in a healthy body, are going to live forever.

No one knows how long life will be. Time is a gift most of us take for granted. Someone living in an unhealthy body has had their future taken away.

They are forced to live in the present. They have also had their purpose taken away. A future and purpose go together. Most of us don't know how to live in the present. We need to help people as they approach the end of their life find a reason to get up in the morning.

SIGNS OF
APPROACHING DEATH

NOTES:

There comes a point in our life, if we are not destined to die a fast death, that our body and living will start to change. Either because of disease or old age, our body will start to release its hold on this earth. Under these circumstances, changes begin to occur between two to four months before actual death from disease. We have already talked about the time difference between disease and old age.

The signs of approaching death from disease are very simple. Months before death, three things begin to occur. Each is on a continuum, changing and increasing as death nears.

Knowing these three things, a person can judge if someone has months, weeks, days or hours to live but we can never be so certain as to be able to put an exact time on death. The dynamics of preparing for death are as varied and individual as the person. Some people will do everything I am going to talk about, some people will do none of the things, but most will exhibit at least some of the signs and dynamics of approaching death.

Months before death occurs from disease, a person's eating habits change. On the continuum, they begin by not eating meat--beef, chicken, fish; then it is fruits and vegetables; then anything that requires energy to digest. After that, the most a person eats is ice cream, puddings, creamed soups, and lastly all they will do is take sips of water.

This is normal and natural. It is how it should be. Yet we have such difficulty when someone is not eating. We can understand that a person is going to die from cancer but it is not okay for a person to starve to death. A person dying from old age or disease does indeed starve to death.

Why do we have so much difficulty with this concept? Food is emotionally intertwined in our lives. We socialize around food. We entertain around food. We use food as an expression of love.

Food is a big part of our holidays. Thanksgiving turkey and all the trimmings, same for Christmas, Easter eggs and chocolate bunnies, 4th of July picnics with fried chicken and corn on the cob, Halloween candy--all food staples of our celebrations.

The real question we need to ask is, why do we eat? The answer is that we eat to live. It is the gas we put in the car to make it run. If the body is preparing to die, it doesn't want the food, it doesn't want the grounding or energy that food brings. The body cuts back on its food intake. It is preparing to let go. Food holds us to this planet.

It isn't that the person doesn't want to eat; they can't

eat. They want to eat for us, their loved ones. They see how important their eating is to us. We'll hear "I can't eat. I put the food in my mouth and it tastes like steel wool. I can't eat."

Unfortunately, a person often gets to the place where they are not taking in enough calories for maintenance and a feeding tube or gastrostomy tube is suggested. When a person has entered the process of releasing from their body and they are not taking enough calories for maintenance, they are weeks from death. When a body is weeks from death nothing works right, every function is starting to shut down. It is not processing. When we feed a person artificially at the end of life, we often end up with more complications than benefits--diarrhea, constipation, aspiration pneumonia.

On this continuum, we reach a place where a person is not taking enough fluids for hydration. This is generally the time intravenous fluids are suggested for hydration. Most people believe that dehydration creates a painful, suffering death. That belief is not true; it is a myth.

If a person has begun the end of life process and they are not taking enough fluids for hydration, they are generally days from death. I've already said their body didn't function properly in the weeks before death when food was an issue. Now, in the days before death, that body is really not working properly. The kidneys are not performing normally, so the fluid that is being forced into the body by way of an IV is not being processed. The body becomes filled with fluid. It feels heavy; sometimes the fluid actually comes out of the tissues. That fluid, not being able to be released from the body, travels up into the lungs and the person drowns.

Visualize a sponge, a dry sponge. Imagine how light

it is. Now in your mind's eye fill that sponge with water. Feel how heavy it has become. That weightiness is the way a body feels when fluid is going in and very little is coming out.

Most people, given a choice, would prefer to die by closing their eyes and just going to sleep. When a person is dehydrated, the electrolytes in their blood stream become abnormal. The calcium elevates. When calcium in the bloodstream becomes too high, a person closes their eyes, goes to sleep and does not wake up. Nature gives us an anesthetic to get through the actual leaving of the body.

The natural way to die from disease and old age is starvation and dehydration. This is a controversial area. For everyone that agrees with this theory you will find the same number that disagrees. (See Interesting Reading at end of book for research materials on this issue.)

At the same time a person's eating habits change, so do their sleeping habits. On a continuum, it starts with taking an afternoon nap, then progresses to a morning and an afternoon nap. Then the person is taking both naps and asleep all evening in front of the television and still sleeps all night. One day they don't get out of bed, they are asleep more than they are awake, and finally they are non responsive.

When a person is asleep more than awake, their reality changes. This world is no longer their reality. The dream world becomes their world. If pain is not an issue, you can wake a person and talk with them. When you leave they will go back to sleep and not know whether they dreamt your visit or if you were really there.

They become confused and disoriented. The veil between the two worlds has thinned so much they are seeing both worlds, this world and the dream world. They are unable to distinguish one from the other.

If I took an 8x10 inch piece of glass and drew a picture on it you could see through the glass and still see the picture. If I drew a different picture on a different 8x10 inch piece of glass and put the two pieces of glass together you would have trouble distinguishing which picture belonged to which piece of glass. The pictures would be superimposed upon each other. That is what happens when a person sleeps more than they are wake. The dream world becomes their reality and this physical world is superimposed upon it.

A person may talk about people and places that make no sense to us. They may talk of a loved one who has already died. Our loved ones who have gone before us come to be with us to help us get from this world to the next.

I have had so many experiences that have convinced me we do not die alone. I will share just two.

I took care of a twenty-three year-old woman. Her primary caregiver was her boyfriend. Three weeks before she died, her brother was killed. Her family chose not tell her he had died. In the week before she died, she started talking to her brother, calling him by name. The boyfriend, thinking she was confused, kept reiterating his name. She finally told him she knew who he was but that her brother was there to help her now.

I also took care of a four year-old that was in the dying process. Both of his parents were already dead. His maternal grandparents were caring for him. In the weeks before he died he told everyone he was taking a trip, that he was going to live with his "parents."

In the hours before his death, he began looking around the room as if searching for something or someone. We asked him what he was doing, and he told us he was looking for his mother. It was as if the room was filled with people we couldn't see. Just before he died, he raised his arm, pointed to the corner of his room and called his mother by name. He stayed focused on that corner until his last breath. You can't convince me his mother wasn't there to help him make the change from this world to the next. We do not die alone!

There is a language that precedes death, a symbolic language. It is often easier to translate that language after death has occurred. "I want to go home," "Get my coat," or another reference to a trip all are signs that death is near.

People in the active role of leaving are like a window into the other world. They tell us what the other

world is like if we will listen to what they are saying.

The third occurrence two to four months before
death from disease is that a person begins to withdraw from the world around them. It begins with a
decreased interest in external matters, sports, the
news, local affairs. On this continuum, it progresses
to not being interested in having visitors, then not
wanting to interact with the family, to completely
withdrawing. It is like they are disconnecting their
threads with people, they are packing their bag of
memories to take with them on their new journey.
This is how it should be. They are letting go of their
hold on this world and building their place in the
other world.

Not always but often a person will actually, in the
weeks preceding death, become hostile and angry,
cutting themselves off from everyone, pushing

everyone away.

If a mother is given a limited prognosis, one begins grieving her death from the moment of her diagnosis. Some days we have her dead and buried and feel very guilty about those thoughts.

Upon diagnosis, the mother is also grieving. She is not only grieving the loss of a daughter, but also the loss of a son, a husband, a job, an identity, a sense of control--the loss of her very life. Something inside of her says, "If I push everyone away now, it won't hurt so much." That isn't true, of course. It hurts terribly. This is when we say, "Mom, I need to be here. I don't know how long we have together. I need every minute I can have with you."

One day my son-in-law brought home one of those fuzzy brown caterpillars you see crawling across the highway. He put it in a glass jar and covered the top with gauze. The caterpillar attached to the gauze and spun a cocoon. We began monitoring that jar, but nothing happened. After several days I got bored, put the jar on the fireplace mantle and promptly forgot about it.

One night I remembered and took the jar down, and there was a beautiful orange and black butterfly inside. We took the butterfly out and as I held it on my finger I had one of those goose bumpy moments that comes in church sometimes. I realized we are all fuzzy caterpillars. If we don't get crushed crossing the highway of life (pardon the pun) then we will withdraw into a symbolic cocoon. It will take us one to three weeks to emerge the beautiful spiritual butterfly that we all are.

In that one to three weeks, family and significant others will get impatient, restless, and will want to get on with their life. We, human beings, can deal with just about any circumstance if we feel the outcome is going to be positive. In our society death is viewed as a negative outcome, so we want the experience to end.

I remember caring for my mother and being frustrated and tired. I just wanted to get on with my life. Immediately I realized in order for me to get on with my life my mother would have to die. Oh, the guilt. It is natural for a caregiver to sometimes feel that we want an end to this experience.

LABOR AND DEATH

NOTES:

There are a lot of similarities between birth and death. Consider a birth into this world as a death in the other world, while a death in this world is a birth into the other side.

We go through labor to get into this world and we go through labor to leave it. The labor to leave this world is harder on us, the watchers, than on the person who is going through the labor. The person who is dying is so removed from their body that they are not experiencing physical sensations in a normal way. Specific physical pain often actually decreases, to be replaced by a heavy all-over ache. At the same time, fear can increase physical pain so we can have a Catch-22 situation.

Some women in labor can sneeze and out pops the baby; other women, thirty-six hours later are still trying to push the little guy out. So it is with the labor to leave this world. Some of us can get out of our bodies more easily than others.

There are three conditions that affect the length of labor to leave this world. One is pain. Physical pain creates a tension that locks us in our body. The key to a gentle death is to relax, to just let go. Physical pain does not allow us to relax. When we alleviate the pain, release can occur.

Fear also creates a tension that locks us in our body and makes our labor longer. Earlier I said we are all going to be afraid to some degree. It is that degree we are concerned about.

Religion can affect our fear of death. If I believe in the concept of Heaven and Hell and also believe that I have not lived up to my religion's expectations of entry into Heaven, then no matter how difficult living is, it does not compare to the idea of eternal damnation. Because we have partial control over the time that we die, we can fight leaving. The fear will create the tension to extend labor.

I took care of a woman who was the most religious person I have ever met. She had the 700 Club on television, all day and night there was gospel music on the radio, the church ladies visited to pray every day, she kept a Bible under her pillow and the minister came several days a week. She didn't die and she didn't die. Her labor went on and on. One day she told me she had done something in her life for which she knew God could not possibly forgive her and that she knew she was going to Hell. I asked if I could talk with her minister about this and was given permission but he could not convince her that God could possibly forgive her. She also gave me permission to have our Hospice Chaplain come and visit. Again she did not feel God could forgive her. She was never going to relax and let go because her fear of punishment and Hell was too great. I think

God finally just said, "Come Mary, come to Me," and took her home.

Unfinished business can make our labor longer. If there is something in my life that I really feel needs to be addressed before I die, with partial control, I can try to stay here until that issue is resolved.

Once, I took care of the perfect family. The adult daughter was the caregiver. She invited her mother and father into her home for the length of her mother's illness. They lived in a perfect house, had perfect children, and she did a perfect job of caring for her mother. But mother just wouldn't let go.

As labor progresses, family members begin to get tired. As we get tired, we can get irritable. When labor goes on and on, families reach a point of exhaustion. With exhaustion we tend to let our barriers down, we become more vulnerable, tempers become less controllable.

So it was with this family. With exhaustion, their defenses came down and one night at the foot of Mom's bed there was a knockdown, drag-out fight between the daughter and her father. All of the past alcoholism, physical and emotional abuse came spewing out--and in the midst of all the clamor, Mom died. The unfinished business was finally addressed.

There is no perfect family. The Cleavers were on television. We are all walking wounded. We are all dysfunctional. It is only a matter of degree that separates us from each other. This is life. There are good times, difficult times, happy times, sad times. It is the name of the game.

Yet we all wear social masks that say we are doing well, that life is as we want it to be. Our job in caring for people at the end of their life is to help them get behind the masks and touch into the wounds so the unfinished business can be addressed.

Earlier I said we couldn't comprehend our own death. There comes a point when a person says, "It's true. They were right. I am going to die." The person knows with the very core of their being that they are going to be dead soon. With this realization, labor begins. They may not share this insight with anyone. They may even deny the knowledge if asked directly, but they know.

The labor to leave this world takes from one to three weeks. The key sign that tells us labor has begun is when a person begins sleeping with their eyes partially open, eyelids at half-mast. It takes energy to keep your eyes open; it takes energy to keep them closed. The normal position for our eyelids is at half-mast.

Other signs are changes in breathing. We may walk into a room, look at the person and think they are not breathing and then, in a short while, they begin taking breaths. Start and stop breathing is an easy way to describe this. They also begin puffing. Their lips are closed and they sort of "blow" out through their lips. Generally they are asleep when doing this.

There comes a general restlessness, agitation, random hand movements, picking of the clothes and bed sheets. This movement can be lack of oxygen but likely also comes from fear. They think that if they lay down and close their eyes they may not open them again. They are right, they may not. They are fighting sleep and they are fighting death.

At this point in the progression towards death, just remember that nothing in the physical body works correctly. The body is shutting down. There is not enough energy or grounding left to maintain functioning. Imagine a light bulb that is not securely fastened into the socket, how it flickers. That is what the physical body is doing now. It is flickering. Sometimes it works, other times not.

Sometimes the body is hot and feverish. Fever in the last weeks or days of life is very common. No need for blood work to be done to find the cause; the cause is approaching death. Cool clothes, acetaminophen, good mouth care, frequent positioning and dry bedding are our healing tools now. We are not trying to "fix" anything. Our goal is to keep the person as comfortable as possible. Our healing work should be focused on healing the emotional, mental and spiritual bodies, not the physical.

Sometimes the body is cold and clammy. Part of the body may be hot, while other parts are cold at the same time. Just remember, nothing works right. The body functions are short-circuiting.

On this continuum, we now approach days to weeks before the actual physical death. Mottling is the key sign for this timeframe. Mottling is the bluish black discoloration of the hands and feet that progresses to a ring around the knees, often with splotches across the back. Mottling is a signal that the body is shutting down.

Mottling is not a signal of approaching death if the person has a heart condition. If heart is not an issue, however, and a person is mottled, then a person has days to a week or so to live.

Mottling is the result of several physical occurrences. A normal blood pressure is 120/80, now the pressure drops to 60/40; maybe there are just a few audible beats at fifty, maybe you can't hear a blood pressure sound at all. That doesn't mean they don't have a blood pressure, it is just so weak you can't hear it.

Our pulse is normally 64-92 beats a minute. Now the pulse is very fast (130-140 beats a minute), weak, and thready. You can feel it by holding the person's wrist, but with difficulty.

We normally breathe 16-24 times a minute. Now breathing is rapid (40-44 times a minute) and shallow. The body is in distress. It is trying very hard to keep working. To help decrease the stress the body is experiencing, the heart cuts back circulation of the blood to the arms and legs and concentrates its flow into the vital organs, the heart and brain. That cutback is what causes mottling.

The person is so removed from this world and their body that they begin to lose control of their bladder and bowels. Incontinence is one more sign of letting go.

There are further changes that signify approaching

death. Minutes to hours before death occurs, breathing again changes. Now it slows to six or eight breaths a minute, and then gradually changes to "fish" breathing. Just picture a fish as it opens and closes its mouth. A person breathes like a fish just before death occurs. That is what the man was doing on the television documentary, and that was what the bird was doing; all of God's creatures breathe like a fish breathes just before they die. They may breathe like that for just one or two breaths, or they may breathe like that for hours. Breathing like a fish is the way we die, fast or gradual death.

A person is also non-responsive. They may be moving about in bed, they may be talking (probably not making sense), but they don't respond to the world around them. You call their name or touch the person and they don't respond. Most of us sleep through our change from this world to the next.

Often in the twenty-four to thirty-six hours before death, a person will appear to rally. They have been in labor for days or weeks and for no apparent reason they wake up and have energy. They may request food and eat it, even visit with friends and family. This is the miracle for which we have all been praying. We think our loved one is going to get well after all. Everyone once again has hope. Then the brief moment is gone and death arrives.

Could it be that we get extra spiritual energy to make the transition from this world to the next? That some of it lapses over into this physical world, giving us the gift of interaction one more time? I like to think that is the explanation for this unusual burst of energy.

In the moments just before death, a phenomenon occurs. Many of us witnessing this occurrence relate it to the specific peculiarities of the person dying, when in fact most people do something of this nature just before death.

Visualize a person, breathing very slowly, like a fish, non-responsive, eyes partially open. They suddenly open their eyes, move their arms or legs, maybe sit up in bed. This last movement is often not so dramatic. Generally there is a slow movement of an arm or shoulder, a gradual frown or grimace on the face. It is almost like a person is saying, "No, I don't want to leave that which I know." This movement is followed by one or two long, spaced-out breaths. You think there will be no more breathing, and there is a gasp.

I believe that the frown or grimace is the actual moment that the "driver gets out of the car," and the last breath or two is just the rest of the air leaving the body.

Know that a person can hear even in the moments following death. Ideally we have taken the opportunity a disease offers us to talk openly with our departing loved one about the effect they have had on our life. Even if we have had this opportunity, it is still good to talk to them again while they are non-responsive. It is a lot easier to talk with someone who is non-responsive, someone who will not argue back.

Talk about the good times and the difficult times. The person who is leaving this world began processing their life months ago. On many different levels of consciousness they asked themselves what their life has been about, whom they have touched and what they have accomplished. Life is like a billion piece jigsaw puzzle, and as we leave this world we try to put all the pieces together in some kind of order, to make some sense of our life.

There is no perfect relationship. If we can tell our loved one how they have affected our life, positively and negatively, we can help them sort out the pieces of their puzzled life. We can also use this opportunity to tell them how much we love them, how much we will miss them, and give them permission to go.

Remember, a person has partial control over the time that they die-- so telling a person they can leave when they are ready helps them address the ambivalence that is present as they begin the final separation from their body. We will try to stay in this world for those we love.

It will never be acceptable for someone that I know and love to die. We will always want them on earth with us. We do not have to tell our loved one it is "okay" for them to die. We can, however, say to them that we understand it is time for them to leave and they can go whenever they are ready.

One day, when I was sixteen and a nurse's aide in a small hospital, the Head Nurse asked me to sit with a patient. She walked with me into a single room that had the lights out and the shades drawn. There, alone in the room, was an unconscious woman. The Head Nurse said to tell her when the woman was dead. She then walked out of the room and closed the door.

I was so frightened. I'd had no experience with dying before, but being the adaptive child that I was, I stayed in the room and did what I was told. I remained as far away from the woman as possible. When my eyes adjusted to the darkness of the room, I could see the woman's chest moving up and down. When I could hear over the pounding of my own heart, I could hear her breathing. I just stood and watched. I don't know how long I was there, but eventually I couldn't hear or see her breathing. I decided that must mean the woman was dead. The Head Nurse confirmed that indeed she had died.

20 some years later, when I was taking a refresher course in nursing, I was working on the oncology floor. The Head Nurse, knowing I was going to work in hospice, took me into a patient's room one day and said, in front of an unconscious woman, "She is dying. You can do anything you want" and left the room, shutting the door.

The room was a single room, lights out, shades drawn, and the woman was alone. I felt a sense of deja vu, and hadn't realized until then what a profound effect the sixteen year-old experience had had on my life. I had come full circle--only this time I wasn't afraid. I had something to do.

I began stroking Bonnie's arm. She was agitated,

restless, murmuring undistinguishable words. I told her my name, and said that I was a nurse and I was going to help her understand what was happening to her. I told her she was dying, that this is what it is like to die. As I gently stroked her arm, I suggested she would see a light more brilliant than the sun, that the Light was God's Light, and to let it enclose her. She would feel more love and joy than she could imagine.

I told her to be like a log that was floating downstream, to just relax and go with the current. Disregard any sights or sounds other than the Light. If she was frightened, she could calmly ask for help and a Spiritual Being would guide and direct her. I suggested she would see loved ones who had died before her on the periphery, but that right now her work was to go to the Light. She would see the others later.

I reminded her that she was a beautiful child of God. I asked her to forgive herself for any ideas of failure or imperfections, reaffirming to her that she had always done the best she could and that we are far harder on ourselves than God will ever be. I encouraged her to relax and told her she could get out of her body as easily as she could get out of a pair of shoes. Just relax.

Bonnie quieted. Within an hour, she had died a peaceful, gentle death.

When my last child was born, I decided that since I had slept through the first two I would watch this time. During the commotion of the labor pains in the delivery room, I forgot this. Then I heard my doctor saying, "Barbara, you said you wanted to watch, look up into the mirror and watch." Those words helped me focus on what I wanted to do and I saw Jackie being born. Jackie would have been born whether I had watched or not, just as Bonnie would have gone into the Light whether I had been there directing her or not. All I did was help Bonnie focus on her work at hand--releasing her physical body.

In the medical profession we are taught to heal, to fix. Being at the bedside during someone's last moments can be frustrating because it is not a time of fixing. It is a time of feeling helpless. Only one person in the room is working and that is the person working to leave their body and this world. This is the chick breaking out of its shell, the butterfly emerging from its cocoon. This we do alone. This breaking loose is an experience all of us will face. This is very much a part of living.

Now you may be wondering where did this strange woman get all these ideas? There are over eight million people in the United States who have had near death experiences, people who have been declared clinically dead and through the wonders of our modern technology have been revived. These people have said, "When I was dead, I saw all that was going on around me. When I was dead, I heard what everyone was saying. I saw loved ones who were dead. I saw a Light more brilliant than the Sun and in that Light was more love and joy than I have words to describe. I was not afraid. There was a Spiritual presence that guided me. I understood my life, not from a judgmental standpoint but from an understanding of why I did what I did." These people and their near death experiences are telling us what it is like to die if we will listen to them.

TOOLS TO HELP WITH APPROACHING DEATH

FOOD

SLEEP

HOSPITALIZATION/FEAR

OPEN & DIRECT COMMUNICATION

SPIRITUALITY

BONDING

LOVE VS. CARING

REASSURRANCE/REPETITION

PAIN

DR. ELIZABETH KUEBLER-ROSS

SUICIDE

911

FIX-IT PERSONALITIES

POEM

NOTES:

Now that we understand there is a process to approaching death from disease and old age, we can be open to addressing the issues that arise during that time--both for the person approaching death and for the family and significant others.

FOOD

Once the process of separating from the physical body begins, months before actual death occurs, issues of nutrition change. When striving for health, we follow the rules of low cholesterol, low fat, exercise, regulated caloric intake, low salt, minimal sweets. All these rules can be forgotten. The focus now becomes high protein and high calories--protein for building, calories for energy.

If the heart isn't an issue, then ignore the rules for a healthy heart; if the pancreas isn't the issue, ignore the rules for carbohydrates and sweets. The new rule is to eat whatever pleases you, eat often and start taking a protein supplement drink. A person must realize they are eating for two, their body and their disease. The disease eats first and what is left the body gets.

Remember the continuum of withdrawing from foods? Meat; fruits and vegetables; anything requiring energy to digest; puddings, creamed soups, scrambled eggs, ice cream; protein supplement; sips of water. Because the natural direction is decreased food intake, our goal for nutrition is to provide as much quality in as little quantity as possible.

Three meals a day is just too much food at one time for a person in this end of life process to consume. They become defeated before they begin by just looking at "all that food." Six small snacks will go down much better--six high protein, high caloric snacks. Let them eat whatever appeals to them, but put it in the form of frequent small snacks.

Even when the person is still eating a fair amount of good quality food, I recommend beginning to drink some sort of protein supplement. There are plenty of commercial products on the market, or you can make your own. (See resources for recipe.) An entire can of protein supplement will gradually become too much. Divide an eight ounce can in half (four ounces) and give four ounces every two hours from the time the person wakes up in the morning until bedtime; that will probably equal four cans. Four cans of three hundred and fifty calories per can is fifteen hundred calories, enough for maintenance if activity is low. The protein supplement every two hours is in addition to the small, frequent high pro-tein, high caloric snacks.

There will come a point on the continuum when the protein supplement may be the only nutritional intake. That is okay and normal. When a person is letting go of their body they don't want the grounding that food brings, so their body sets the pace without them even realizing it. It is okay that they are not eating, but always offer them food. Let the person make the decision to not eat what is presented.

Again, I stress that part of the normal approach to death from disease or old age is a gradual decrease in food intake. Always offer food, but don't force. By following the above food regime we are only trying to buy time and energy. We will only be successful for a short time. No matter our efforts, the person will eventually stop eating, the body will just refuse to eat or process food. This is normal and natural.

SLEEP

When sleeping patterns change in the months before death we again have to adjust our traditional thinking. Instead of pushing activity, which in a health situation increases strength, we now limit activity to increase strength. Sleep becomes our friend. It recharges our battery and gives us the energy to do what is special for us.

Our body is like a battery that is losing its charge. The closer death approaches, the less "charge" the body has. Our activity level relates directly to how much energy our physical body has left. Sleep "recharges" our body for a time. That length of time is also related to where we are on the continuum of approaching death.

If I want to go to church, I may have to take a nap before I leave and then come home to rest afterward. If the grandchildren are coming over for dinner, I may have to choose between getting out of bed and going to the table or eating in bed with the grandkids sitting with me. Choices of how to spend energy, with sleep as the friend, make activity possible.

HOSPITALIZATION/FEAR

Most hospitalizations in people that can't be fixed are out of fear, not out of need. Often it is fear the caregiver is experiencing as a result of the immense responsibility of caring for a loved one who will die. We put tremendous pressure on caregivers with the medical duties we assign. In the early 1980's I worked very hard to get a patient out of the hospital and home to die. She was receiving an IV of glucose, sugar water. The doctor said he would only let her go home if she had twenty-four hour RN coverage in the home to monitor the intravenous infusion. With much effort, we got the insurance company to agree to pay and the woman went home to die with her IV's and RN's.

Today, it is a whole different scenario. We have patients receiving narcotics intravenously, TPN (balanced nutrition), even blood transfusions all in the home as a matter of routine. We educate the caregiver with hands-on practice, leave an instruction manual detailing the machines, a phone number for emergencies and then leave the family as the caregiver. This is now an acceptable and expected practice. Medical care has come a long way in twenty years, but families are just as scared. They want to do a good job, but are very afraid of doing the wrong thing and hurting their loved one.

Nobody likes to roll out of bed at three in the morning to make a house call, particularly when the medical professional could probably address the situation over the phone. But fear generally needs the physical reassurance of face-to-face support. Fear needs a professional to look at our loved one and say, "This is normal. Everything is going as it should. It is okay." A home visit can neutralize the fear of the caregiver, the fear that they are doing the wrong thing and causing their loved one discomfort. Fear that what is occurring is not "normal," that it is harmful. These are the very reasons hospice policy is to have twenty-four hour on-call service. A big part of the work of hospice is to neutralize the fear that is associated with dying and death; being as close as the phone helps with the neutralization.

OPEN AND DIRECT COMMUNICATION

It is very frightening to be told our loved one "can't be fixed," to be told, "Go home put your affairs in order, you are going to die soon." Because we have no accurate role models, we don't really know what is going to happen or when to expect actual death. Fear walks with us every day. Our imagination, our fantasy of what will happen, becomes far worse than the actual happening. Because of our active imaginations, families need to be told about the dying process. The most frequently asked question from family members is, "How long is it going to be?" We can't be specific when we answer that question, but we can explain the three categories regarding the signs of approaching death and the continuum. Understanding the process and the signs to look for gives a framework which helps neutralize some of the fear the families are facing.

I tell families what to expect because they need the information to begin to prepare themselves for what lies ahead. Many people are uncomfortable with this knowledge. It takes away the illusion that death won't be the end result. Families and significant others do not have to believe what I am telling them but I do make sure they listen to what I have to say. When this difficult time is over they will generally look back and be thankful.

I am not as direct or forceful with the patient. Everyone has the right to be told once they can't be fixed. What they then do with that knowledge is their choice. If they choose to deny the eventuality, that's their choice. It is not up to me to say to them they must believe and deal with their approaching death. Denial may be their only coping mechanism. Some people believe if they talk about death and dying that they will surely die.

I accept a person wherever they are in coping with their diagnosis and terminality. I work with them from that point. I will tell them on our first meeting, during our get acquainted time, that I don't lie, I try very hard not to play games, and I will talk about anything. I also say there are signs I look for that tell me if a person has months, weeks, days or hours to live and if they ever want to know what those signs are, just ask me. This way I have not told them something they are not ready to hear, but have left the door open for them when they are ready.

Selective hearing enters into play here also. We tend to hear only what we want to hear. I am open and honest, but gentle and very tactful. If a person in denial is talking unrealistically about their future or capabilities, I will not agree with them. An example is my exchange with a gentleman I'll call Bill who was very much in denial. "He was going to beat this thing." I would find him on my visits sitting in a chair in front of his fireplace, golf polyesters on, little alligator on his shirt, smiling his skeletal smile. It took him all morning to get up and dressed for the day and then he slept most of it in the chair. One day he said his friend had given him a set of golf clubs, and when he was at the doctor's office that week he had asked the doctor if he should keep the clubs, so he could play golf in the spring. It was January. The doctor told him, of course, to keep the clubs; he would be on the course in the spring.

Bill looked me in the eye and said, "What do you think?" This was during the time that I still used the word terminal. My reply was, "We both know you have a terminal illness. No one knows how long someone has to live, but Bill, this is probably as good as it is going to get." His response to my directness was that I was the first person who had ever used the word "terminal" in reference to his condition, except for himself.

Something interesting transpired here. In order to be on hospice, Bill had been told by his physician he couldn't be fixed. He was also told that hospice cares for people with a six-month prognosis and signed Medicare papers stating the same. He just wasn't ready or willing to cope with that kind of knowledge.

We generally don't ask a question of this nature unless we have the answer somewhere inside. By not telling the truth when asked, we destroy any kind of trust we may have been establishing. Bill had come to terms, his own terms, with his prognosis. He knew the answer before he asked the doctor if he should keep the golf clubs. It was a test and the doctor failed. Bill was opening the door now to talk about his end of life issues. By not pushing him, yet building a relationship and bond with him, we reached a place of trust and we talked.

SPIRITUALITY

Just as we should accept a person for where they are with their coping skills, we should accept their belief system. The bedside is not the place to share our personal religious theories. If someone believes that pink elephants are going to get him or her through the night, then support them in that idea. "Saving" a person is left to invited clergy, no one else.

I took care of a father-daughter family. The daughter called hospice and said she would like hospice services for her father, but they were both atheist-- and if we were going to sell any "God Crap" (her words not mine), then she didn't want us. I assured her I didn't have to talk about God to provide hospice care. I was their primary care nurse for three months. One day the father asked me what I believed happened when someone died. I shared my belief with him. His response was he hoped that was the way it was going to be. After I left, I immediately called the daughter and told her about the conversation. She replied she just wanted whatever her father wanted and was appreciative that I had told her of the conversation. I know beyond a doubt if that situation had occurred three days or three weeks after hospice services began, I would have been accused of "selling God crap." Because I'd had three months to build a relationship based on trust, the exchange had a positive ending. I don't know what I would have said if he had asked that question earlier in our relationship, but I guarantee the response from the daughter would have been negative.

"The rest of the story" is that at the visitation, the casket was placed by the funeral home under a very large picture of Jesus praying in the garden of Gethsemane. The daughter was very upset, so the two of us took down the picture and placed it in the back hall. Instead of a traditional religious service, there were individual readings of poetry and prose, personal sharing, and much love, caring and support throughout. Not one word of God was spoken, yet from someone who comes from a God base, I felt more spirituality in that room then I have felt in many a church. If God is Love, then God was present for that family.

Sometimes we let our preconceived ideas of tradition and acceptability get in the way of just being present and experiencing a non-distorted moment.

Because we tend to associate death with "meeting our Maker," we ascribe a religious theme to end of life issues. Religion may be there for many of us, but we must remember religion is not a part of everyone's daily life. If prayer has not had a prominent place in a person or family's life, it will not necessarily have meaning at the end of life. Remember, we die the way we have lived. If we have not turned to a minister, priest or rabbi for comfort in other challenging times, most likely we will not do it now.

I have seen many a priest or clergyperson called to the bedside of a person dying or who has just died. Most bring comfort and support, but how ineffectual are the few who enter, say a few prayers and leave. Where is the comfort in a few prayers? A touch, a sincere presence with no words, has more comfort than prayers without personal interaction. During a time of great loss, personhood is the most meaningful and healing.

BONDING

In our society there is an unspoken ritual for getting acquainted with another person. It begins with small talk, and gradually over a period of time and meetings we reveal more of ourselves to each other. We test the waters for acceptance and rejection as we allow the layers of our personality to be seen.

In working with someone who has a limited prognosis, time is the enemy. There is not time for the social ritualizing often needed to become a trusted friend. That ritual could take weeks, even months. Here are some simple ideas that work on a subconscious level to speed up the bonding process.

If you are a professional, church member, lay minister or volunteer, always wear your nametag. There is so much stress and so many people that are in and out of a family's life that it is impossible to remember everyone by name. By wearing a nametag, you are allowing the other person the dignity of not having to ask your name.

When I arrive for the first meeting, I introduce myself using my first and last name and I shake hands. Shaking hands is a socially acceptable way to touch. Touch helps us bond with one another.

I ask permission to call everyone by their first name. It is hard to be open with the formality of "mister" or "missus". Different cultures have different approaches to the use of those titles. Know and respect the culture.

Studies have been done about the perception of standing verse sitting while talking. Sitting conveys the idea of unhurried friendliness. Staying below the other person's eye level also removes a distance between people. Sit at eye level or below when conversing. Putting this in practice means I have spent many a conversation sitting on the floor next to a person sitting in the chair. Being on the floor also gives the impression of informality and closeness. This is done when there are no close chairs available. I also ask permission to sit on the bed. Pain may be an issue, yet the person may not feel at ease enough to protest the invasion of their bed space. Asking allows them the opportunity to say no.

I sit as close to the people I am talking to as possible without being invasive. When I enter a home to talk with a patient and the spouse, and the patient is sitting on the sofa, I will choose the sofa to sit on also. If the patient is in a chair, I will find the closest chair in which to sit or I will sit on the floor. If we are sitting at a table, I will choose a chair next to the patient rather than be across from him and have the table between us. I want to be able to reach out and touch when we are talking about sensitive areas. I do not touch a person immediately if they are crying. Touch often hinders the expression of emotions, so I will be close and supportive but not touch for a while.

There are people who are comfortable with touch and those that are not. Watch body language to guide you in the effort to touch another. I am a hugger of people, that is who I am, but I don't hug without asking permission first. I literally say, "I am a hugger, may I give you a hug?" That said, I watch for body language as I approach. Some people are comfortable with front-on hugs; others will give permission but are not so sure and will turn sideways. A sideways turner gets an arm around the shoulder kind of hug. Whatever the kind of touch, it is one step toward getting closer quicker.

Another way of getting closer is to speak plain English as opposed to medicalese. As I said earlier, people under stress do not have the energy to translate what you are saying. They will listen and nod, but generally not tell you they don't have a clue about what you are telling them. Even if a person has a PhD, this is not the time to expect them to understand medical terminology. Don't talk down to them, but be sure to speak slowly and clearly, using a vocabulary that is simple enough to be grasped immediately.

LOVE VS. CARING

As we work closely with people, we often find some individuals who become more special to us than others. Most times, people I am involved with I see as children of God. Every so often, a person becomes more than that to me. I care for them as people special to Barbara. These feelings are generally reciprocal and as the relationship develops, words are exchanged as to how meaningful the relationship has become. The relationship goes from professional to personal.

I learned early on the ramifications of using the word love when talking about feelings for another. Most people do not take the meaning of the word love much further than romantic love. It can really confuse the boundaries to say, "I love you" to a patient or any person you are working with on a professional level. We may really be saying, "You have become very special to me as a person," but what is actually heard is sometimes misunderstood. It is much less confusing to either just say, "You have become very special to me" or "I care about you very much." There is no gray area about the word "caring"; no misunderstanding can come from that phraseology.

REASSURANCE/REPETITION

Families and significant others need continuous reassurance and repetition. Under stress, our memories fail. If you want someone to remember something, write it down for them. Make written care plans that outline when medicines are to be given, treatments administered, when voiding and bowel movements occur, and what kind of activities were performed. Make a list for water and food intake. A caregiver is not going to remember any of the above, and that is all information medical professionals need to know to evaluate their patient's condition.

I used to leave a home and think I sounded like a broken record; repeating and repeating, visit after visit, but that was the only way to insure a family learned what I was teaching them. The retention level for people under stress is almost nonexistent. Repeating and writing insures the family and significant others have the skills to provide good home care.

Reassurance is very important also. We all blossom with praise. It makes us strive to do even better. It builds self-confidence. Reassurance is given to not only the family and caregivers, but to the patient. It is hard work to be sick. It requires a great deal of patience and courage. It is helpful to acknowledge with praise the difficult life work that is being done. Just opening their eyes each day requires bravery. When we recognize that bravery we give strength to face the challenge of being alive.

PAIN

Pain management and medications are such a rapidly changing area that if I were to write about specific drugs, they would probably be obsolete by the time this book is published. But I will discuss a few principles that no matter the rapidly changing venue will probably stay the same.

If you and I have a headache, we can each take two aspirin and the headaches will probably go away. No matter our relative sizes, two aspirin will probably do the trick. Not so with pain medications. Each person's pain and discomfort is different. Our levels of pain tolerance are individual. The reason for our pain, even for those people with the same disease, is not going to be the same. Body size, weight, age, location of the tumor or disease condition, and even treatment factors all contribute to the intensity of physical pain. Fear, no matter its origin, also increases physical pain. All of these different factors mean that an across the board dosage of any particular pain medicine is inappropriate. A professional in pain management, cancer pain in particular, must find the correct dosage to fit the specific pain pattern of an individual. It may take days before sufficient pain management is reached. This is generally done by gradually increasing the dosage of the chosen drug.

Using the aspirin analogy again, if I take those two aspirin for my headache, the headache will probably go away and not return until a cloudy day or I get stressed again. With the pain from cancer, the pain medication does not make the pain "go away" like the aspirin did for the headache. The pain medicine merely covered the pain; the cause is still there and will return when the medicine leaves the body. Pain medication, for cancer pain in particular, must be taken on an around the clock, continued basis. This is done whether the pain is being experienced or not. If the pain is gone, that means the medicine is working. To stop taking the medication only removes the continued presence of the "cover" and the pain will return. This is very important! I can't tell you how many times people have stopped taking the pain medication because they were not hurting, only to be surprised when the pain returned.

Our drug environment today has made us very aware of the dangers of taking narcotics. Most of my patients were concerned about taking medicines for pain in the fear of becoming addicted and/or of overmedicated. Actually, it is very difficult to overdose and die from a narcotic we have been taking routinely. The signs of overdosing are drowsiness, thick tongue, slurred speech, seeing things that aren't there, confusion and slowed breathing, generally in that order. When those signs begin to occur, we simply don't take the next scheduled medication dosage and call hospice or our medical professional for adjustments to be made to the medication. Drowsiness, however, can occur simply because a person is exhausted and now that they are more comfortable, they can sleep.

There is a thin line in our body between pain and no pain. It is that line that a professional is trying to reach in good pain management. Addiction occurs when there is consistently more pain medicine in the body than pain. The person on the street who puts a narcotic into their system and has no pain issues is the one that becomes addicted. Pain management is administering the appropriate level of medicine to match the present pain. There will be no danger of addiction or overdosing when delivered properly.

Pain is a very difficult occurrence to assess. If you see my arm is hanging at an odd angle and I say it is painful, you can see the source of the pain and will probably believe me. But most pain is not visible. Most pain is subjective. If I tell someone that I hurt very badly, even if I say on a scale of one to ten this is a ten, that person just has to believe me. I may have nothing to "show" for my pain. Also what is a ten to me may be a five to someone else. What is important here is that a ten is a ten if the person thinks it is. Pain is what I, the one hurting, say it is, not what an observer thinks it should be.

Physical pain is like living behind a large brick wall. A person can't see anything but the pain. Maslow's Theory is that there is a hierarchy of needs beginning with the physical, progressing to emotional, mental, and spiritual. The essence of Maslow's Theory is that you can't talk about emotional issues if someone is in physical distress. Remove the physical obstacles first and progress to the others in due time.

DR. ELIZABETH KUEBLER-ROSS

Dr. Elizabeth Kuebler-Ross talked about the five stages that a person experiences when approaching death: denial, bargaining, anger, depression and acceptance. She has clarified the progression of these five stages. The word stages seems to imply that having gone through one, you move on to the next, that there is completion of one before moving on. Not so. A person can be angry about their prognosis and five minutes later be in denial of even having a limited prognosis. There is no completion. There is no time frame. There is a continued experience of these feelings until withdrawal and sleep have consumed the ability to care.

Denial is a coping life skill. If I deny the existence of a situation, then I don't have to take responsibility for addressing the outcome. After all, if something doesn't exist; I don't have to deal with it. Remember, we will cope with the challenge of dying in the same manner we cope with other life occurrences. Denial may be our only way "to get through the night." I don't take that away from people. Others may disagree with my approach.

Anger is a very normal reaction to the news of a life threatening illness and limited prognosis. If someone were pleased with the news, that would be abnormal. Anger is difficult because it is hard to direct. Are we angry with ourselves, God, the doctors, nurses and/or hospital? We may be angry with all of the above, but the real issue of the anger is that we are going to die; our life is coming to an end.

That abstract concept provides no place to "put" our anger. We, Americans, are a blaming society. We want to blame someone or something for our death sentence, so that means we need a hook on which to place our anger. God, ourselves, the doctors, nurses and/or hospital offer that hook. Being angry applies not only to the patient but family and significant others as well.

When we become angry with ourselves, we generally don't talk about it but hold the anger inside. It has no outlet when held inward and becomes depression.

Again, depression is a normal, natural aspect of coping with a life threatening illness--whether it's ours or someone else's. If someone is jumping for joy, there is something wrong with them. It is very sad to consider leaving family, friends, our very life. Unfortunately, we are often in too big of a hurry to get rid of the depression so we resort to antidepressant medication. We rush to cover up the sad feelings rather than use the opportunity to look at our life, to feel our emotions.

Our dying experience can be our most glorious moment, a time when we do the best work of our life. Some people never really live until they have been told they are going to die. For others, dying will be the most terrifying time of their life. The choice of how we approach this final challenge is entirely up to us. Depression and how we manage our feelings is part of that work.

I am not saying there is no place for antidepressants. Sometimes people get in such a deep, dark hole they need medication to bring them up to the surface so they can do their final work. I am saying that we tend to rush into medications too quickly in most cases.

Acceptance implies comfort with a situation. In this case, that it is all right to die. It will never be "okay" to die, not for myself or any one close to me. I will always want that person physically with me. Few people reach the place of acceptance. I would like to substitute the word understanding for acceptance. It is very possible to reach a place of understanding: understanding that I am going to die, understanding that my loved one is going to die. I don't want it to happen, but I understand it will.

SUICIDE

Before I began working for hospice, I took a course in crisis and suicide intervention. I thought working in hospice I would see a lot of suicides. I was so wrong. In the twenty plus years of working in hospice, I can count on one hand the number of patient suicides or even attempts that I've encountered. What I did witness was that most people diagnosed with a life threatening illness think about suicide. It is a normal and natural thought process.

What thinking about suicide in this situation really shows is that we are probably more afraid of the experience of dying than of actually being dead. It is getting there that is so scary, the fear of pain, dependency, loss of control, all of those issues that will affect us as death approaches. The response to those fears is to bypass the experiences and die right now.

What keeps us from doing that is most of us do not have the courage to kill ourselves. It is easy to think about but it is very hard to do. Most of us are not emotionally strong enough to end our life. That is why we want assisted suicide laws, why we ask others to help us. If we were able to do it ourselves, we wouldn't need to ask others.

When I approach a person who has spoken to me about suicide, I first reassure them I am not going to place any judgment on them for having those thoughts, that those thoughts are normal for the life situation they are currently facing. I help them explore why they want to end their life now and address the issues raised. Generally the issues are about fear, as mentioned earlier, of pain, dependency and loss of control.

I am making this sound very simple, but it isn't. It takes patience, tact, teaching, listening, and a wide variety of skills that I can't impart in these few pages. I do want to say that one of the things I stress is for people not to ask someone to help them take their life. Aside from the fact you are putting the other person in an illegal situation, most people are not emotionally equipped to live with the knowledge that they helped kill another human being.

911

We have been conditioned to believe if we call 911,

help will arrive. For a medical emergency, para-medics will come and rescue us from our difficulty. For someone with a life threatening illness, some-one who has entered the dying process, this isn't necessarily true. In fact, calling 911 can be a detri-ment.

If I stick my finger in a light socket and my heart stops, I want someone to give me CPR and call 911. When the paramedics arrive, they will probably be able to start my heart and I will return to my normal life and activities. If my body is filled with cancer, kidney or liver failure, or AIDS; if I've had a serious stoke from which there is no rehabilitation potential; if the doctors have said they can't fix me and my heart stops and you call 911 or I don't have a signed Do Not Resuscitate form in a hospital or nursing facility, some medical person is going to try to start my heart. They may succeed. I have seen it happen many times. BUT they will still not be able to fix the cancer, the AIDS, the kidney or liver failure or the stroke that I died from in the first place. I will just have to die again in a short time. I, personally, would not be happy with anyone that did that to me. Most people wouldn't.

I took care of an elderly couple that were on the brink of refinancing their home. They needed money to pay for the continued medical expenses of the 76 year old husband. He had been coded in the hospital on one of his many readmissions for cancer of the head and neck. At the time of his code, he had a gastrostomy, could not talk, was bedfast, sleeping most of the time and only semi-alert. He had entered the dying process. But instead of letting that natural process occur, someone tried to "fix" him. They stopped his dying, for the moment, but did not "fix" his quality of life. He was still unable to communicate, had a gastrostomy, was bedfast and now only barely alert. He was sent home with his wife, his only caregiver. She couldn't care for him though, because she was in her 70's and in ill health herself. Hospice was called in, and an anguishing pain-filled month later, the gentleman died. This is just one of many similar stories I could tell.

FIX-IT PERSONALITIES

If, as caregivers, we are spending more time and energy trying to solve a family's particular problem than the family, then that family is comfortable with their problem and does not have the desire to solve the situation. The question becomes, "Who wants the problem solved?" Sometimes we, as caregivers, identify a life challenge in other's lives and deem it needs adjusting. From our perspective, from our personal lives, the difficulty may indeed need fixing; it becomes the "I couldn't live like that" syndrome. What we need to remember is the family can and is "living like that." This lifestyle, whatever the degree of dysfunction, is meeting their needs if they are not anxious to change it. The tumultuous time of coping with the approaching death of a loved one (or disliked one) is generally not the time people are receptive to changing patterns that have taken a lifetime to create.

It is important to help the patient and family draw on their own skills and coping mechanisms. We fix-it personalities (volunteers, medical and service-oriented professionals tend to be fix-it personalities) want to take over a situation and fix it for another. It is a big trap into which we often fall. A person is floundering in their life challenge; we rush in, take it on and try to resolve everything for them. The question then becomes, who learned from the challenge? The person to whom life presented that challenge? I think not. We can support, nurture, and offer guidance and options, but it is not for us to take over.

Many times I see people very frustrated because those involved in what we consider "dysfunctional behavior" are not attempting to find solutions. When an outsider is spending more energy trying to "fix" a challenge than the person who is challenged, then it is the outsider that wants it fixed. Many people are very comfortable in what appears discomfort to someone else. Again, we can support, nurture, offer guidance and options, avoid game-playing, get anyone out of harm's way that needs it, and administer our particular skills. Then go home at night knowing we have completed a day of good work.

One day I visited with a woman patient, my age. She had children similar ages to myself. We talked for several hours about her anger, that because she would soon be dead she would never see her daughters graduate from high school, attend their weddings or see her grandchildren,. She was so angry at her fate, at being robbed of what she had expected from life. She raged, cried, sobbed and at last just lay spent in my arms.

When I left her house I felt good. I had accomplished something important.

From her home I drove to a hospital to visit another patient. Following that visit, while still in the parking lot, I sat in my car and cried. There was no satisfaction, no sense of accomplishment, only frustration with human carelessness. I pulled out a piece of paper and wrote the following. I share it here as a tool to aid in keeping a clear perspective on working with end of life issues.

I work with dying people, all my patients die.
I see grief and sadness and anger and depression.
Most is an individual's internal anguish needing to
    be brought out, to be worked out.
Nowhere is it written that life will always be the
    way we'd like it to be.
Dying presents us with perhaps the greatest oppor-

tunity for growth we have ever had.
This struggle is part of life; it is a learning process-
Learning to live
Learning to die
That is what physical life is all about.
There is no pain for me here.

Today I walked into a hospital room.
My patient/friend was strapped in a wheelchair,
Facing a blank wall,
His back turned to a blaring TV and the door,
His body heavy and uncomfortable falling limply
    over the side of the chair,
His arm blue from hanging too long a time at his
    side.
Unable to talk because of a brain tumor,
Unable to maneuver his body,
He was trapped by someone else's hurriedness.
Poop on his hands, from poop in his pants,
He took my hand in his and kissed it--
A thank you for getting him back into bed
And my heart cried.
Here lies my pain!
The indignities that need not be in life for lessons to
    be learned,
The indignities imposed upon man by man,
Here in lies my pain!

TIME OF DEATH

NOTES:

The approaching death of someone we care about is very, very sad. But while it is never all right for someone we know and love to die, that experience does not have to be bad. There are two times that we are closest to God: when we leave home and when we return home; when we are born and when we die. If we can get beyond our fears, we can touch the spirituality of the moment. Fear blocks us from experiencing the beauty of being present during the final life experience. Everyone dies. It is an important life moment for all of us. Sharing that moment is a very special gift.

As we said in Chapter One, we have partial control over the time that we die. None of the dying process is accidental. We have control, even though it appears to the contrary. When the end stage of labor to leave this world continues into a week or two and unfinished business, pain and fear have been addressed, realize that someone is learning something. There is some dynamic occurring that is necessary before the person can leave their body. This is the time faith plays a big part for the family and significant others. Faith that all is as it should be, that nothing bad is happening, that for some the process to leave the body is more difficult than for others.

We in the medical profession have not really been taught about caring for someone during the final time of living. We are taught to heal, to fix, to cure. Attention is not placed on what to do when our efforts fail. No one is bold enough to say that at some point death becomes the goal--a gentle, peaceful, natural death. Dying from disease or old age goes against everything medical professionals have learned, so we often come empty-handed to the bedside when death will be the eventual outcome. Family and significant others come empty-handed also because they lack proper role models.

A death from disease or old age is not a physical event. It is a social event. During the labor to leave the body, those minutes to hours, even days before death, the physical body has no demands other than cleanliness and comfort. Cleanliness is frequent mouth and eye care, appropriate changing of diapers and bed linen. It is the inserting of a catheter to eliminate the discomfort of being in a wet bed. It is wiping the face and body if clammy and damp.

Comfort is scheduled positioning, good skin care and maintaining pain management. It is not frequent blood pressure checks or invasive procedures. If there is a blood pressure reading of 60/40 or just a few beats at 50, repeated taking of the blood pressure just points to the need of the professional to do something, not to gathering pertinent information. The same is true with a minimal pulse.

How hydrated or dehydrated a person is will determine how much and how loud their congestion will be. A suction machine is generally not beneficial at this time. It simply irritates the throat, pulls out existing oxygen and actually triggers the body to produce more secretions. Often times repositioning the person to a side will lessen the sound of the breathing. Most important is to tell those present what is happening and why. Congestion is a part of the dying process. It often happens when death approaches. It is not bad. It is natural and normal.

Once a person is actively dying, address the needs of the family and significant others. Assist them in talking with the non-responsive patient. Help neutralize the fears that each person is bringing to the deathbed. Explain to those present what is happening and what will happen, what they will see as death approaches and breathing stops. We can deal with anything if we know what to expect. It is our fantasy that is far worse than reality.

During those waiting hours encourage the family to share life stories, look at family albums and photographs, reminisce. A lighted candle and/or the playing of favorite music also enhance the feeling of love and beauty and help neutralize fear.

There is no need for darkened rooms, pulled shades or the person to be alone. A quiet gathering of family and friends to say goodbye is needed here. Crying is very acceptable; after all, we are sad that someone we care about is leaving. Each culture has its own approach to emotions, with none being right or wrong. This is a time of saying goodbye. Forever partings are difficult to take. Remind those present that the person is preparing to leave this world. They are working to exit their cocoon of a body. Respect and reverence needs to be shown during this time.

Nurses frequently ask, "What do I do when I have never met the family and I am called to a situation where the patient is actively dying? What do I do and say?" First and foremost, be yourself. Bring who you are, sincerely, into the situation. Assess what is occurring; determine who is present and how everyone is coping. Then proceed to educate in a gentle, nurturing way. Remember, everyone there is bringing their perceived ideas of what this death will be like, they are all emotionally involved and they are frightened. They need to know what to expect. Proceed as if they know nothing about the dying process, as if no one has given them any preparation.

It helps if you have knowledge of the particulars of the family psychosocial history, religious affiliation and diagnosis, but it isn't necessary. You can ask questions of those present if there is something you feel you need to know. The bottom line is, if you have determined the person is in labor and has minutes to hours to live, help those present say goodbye.

You can be a nurse, a social worker, a member of the clergy, a lay minister or a next-door neighbor and be an excellent guiding force. Remember, this is a social occurrence not a medical event.

The last moments before death are a time of great feelings of helplessness. However, there is healing work to be done, and just not physical healing work. Encourage all present to say goodbye, alone, in their special way. Then, as the breathing slows and the fish breathing begins, gather around the bed. Tell everyone the time has come; you think the person is leaving now. Watch for the grimace and subtle movement. When that occurs, tell everyone there will be just a few more breaths as the rest of the air leaves the body. I generally stand at the side of the head of the bed with my fingers placed in the space between the collarbone and the neck. With practice you can feel the release of the body, when there will be no more breaths. If you are not part of the family or significant others then you want to be as invisible as possible. Yet you can still be a guide much like a conductor leading an orchestra.

When you are sure there will not be another breath, there is really no need to get out a stethoscope if you are a medical person. To be blunt, dead is dead, and you can tell. Before you call the funeral home, tidy the body, remove the catheter, wash any soiled body areas. It is not necessary to give the body a complete bath; however, in assessing family members, having them help with a final bath can be a great tool for diminishing guilt and easing grief. Put on a low light, straighten the room, put the side rails down, put on a clean gown if the current one is soiled, do the same thing with the sheets or blanket. Elevate the head of the bed, if it is a hospital bed, just enough so the body looks natural and position the head with pillows if necessary. You are trying to get the body in a natural position. This is the last time those present will see their loved one in a natural setting and you want to create a comforting memory.

Now that a positive scene is set, encourage each person to go back into the room and say goodbye again to their loved one. This is the last natural contact they will have with the person they care about. Suggest that they say aloud or in their mind whatever is in their heart about the person who has just died.

When everyone has had an opportunity to say goodbye, and that includes Aunt Bertha from across town, explain that you will call the funeral home. While waiting, you may talk about plans for the visitation and funeral, about whom they are going to notify by phone, about what the funeral home people will do when they arrive at the house.

It is often more comfortable if everyone wait in another room while the body is put on the gurney for removal from the house. Ask if they want the face covered or uncovered, and if they would like to walk the body to the car. Those are all choices most people don't know they can make.

When the funeral home personnel arrive, I go into the room with them as a family representative. As soon as the body is out of the bed, even while the funeral home people are arranging the body on the gurney, I lower the head of the bed, straighten the sheets and pillows, and make the bed as I would if I had a bedspread. I then look for something to put on the pillow--a flower, a picture, a Rosary, a Bible, a stuffed animal, anything to make the bed seem less empty. Imagine how difficult it is to return to a room where someone you care about has died. By not leaving a stark, empty, unmade bed, we are creating a small memorial space. Leave a low light on when you leave the room. Again think how unpleasant it would be to have to enter a darkened room.

LIVING WITH A
LIFE THREATENING
ILLNESS

NOTES:

In 18 months between 1993 and 1995, my mother and stepfather were both diagnosed with cancer of the lung. Our experience--theirs as people living with a life threatening illness, and mine as a relative and caregiver--taught me about dealing with illness. As a caregiver my perception was subjective, as opposed to the objective viewpoint of a nurse. That 18 month period gave me invaluable firsthand knowledge which, when I was able to distance myself emotionally a year later, added to my empathy and understanding of the feelings of those living with illness. No amount of reading, study or workshops could have taught me what I will share here. This becomes an overview of caregiver and patient experience from the knowledge base of a trained hospice professional who became a personal caregiver.

A little background information: my mother's name is Dorothy and my stepfather is Don. They were both in their 70's when they died. They both were smokers for many years. Don was diagnosed with Oat Cell cancer of the lung, a very fast-growing, seldom fixable kind of cancer. Prognosis is generally four to six months, depending upon when it is discovered. Dorothy's cancer was Sequamous cell, a slow-growing, non-fixable cancer. Prognosis is generally undeterminable. Radiation may alleviate some symptoms.

Dorothy was diagnosed in spring of 1993 and died eighteen months later in February of 1995, having had no treatment for her cancer. Don was diagnosed in the spring of 1994 and died four months later in September of 1994. He chose to have intensive chemotherapy and radiation. Within 5 months of each other, both of my parents were dead.

Each chose their own unique course toward the end of life. My mother accepted the situation and looked for quality time. She probably did her finest work in those eighteen months before her death. My stepfather chose to deny even a hint that the treatment might not be successful. It seems to me his last months were a waste, with energy spent on a "cure" that only his oncologist, radiologist and he believed in. Time was spent in doctors' offices, laboratories, treatment rooms, hospitals and home in bed. Time was spent experiencing all the debilitating side effects of high dose chemotherapy and radiation; it was not spent experiencing the joys of what was left of a life.

DIAGNOSIS ISSUES

From the moment a physician says the dreaded words, "You have cancer," life will never be the same. Ever! Oh, we want it to be, we fantasize about when it was "normal," but life changes in that millisecond and can never be recovered.

Normalcy is gone and replaced with illness. Simple conversation styles are changed. Instead of "What are you doing?" the first question becomes "How are you?" Instead of talking about the weather or adventures or just gossipy things, conversations center around the illness and physical body issues. It seems as though the spontaneity of life has diminished. The laughter, jokes, the joys of life are harder to come by. They are there, but are hidden by the dark cloud of an uncertain future. The thought "cancer," and all that word denotes, hovers unspoken, always.

Normalcy is replaced by uncertainty and fear. Our life becomes the unknown. In reality it has always been an unknown, but we live under the illusion we have control of our environment. That illusion has been destroyed along with so many other beliefs.

We feel unsteady; not only do we feel physically

unwell, but emotionally and mentally we are also suffering.

There are so many questions but very few answers. We even question the questions. Should we ask? Do we really want to know? Are we being told the "truth?" Our mind isn't as clear as it once was. We need to think, to make decisions, but we just don't seem to have the strength. It is easier to just go along with whatever the doctors and health care professionals say. "They are the experts, after all. Let them fix me." Our decreased physical capacity affects our mental abilities. Unfortunately, this is at a time when we need all the clarity we can muster.

Uncertainty about what the future holds is ever-present. What does a person do when there is no future to look forward too? How do we cope when the future only holds possible pain, loss and death? Fear becomes a constant companion.

The future becomes so frightening it becomes worse than the fear of being dead. At least when you are dead you don't hurt, you don't feel, the nightmare is over. Depression and thoughts of suicide play with our mind.

Our thoughts of uncertainty turn to others in our life, those we have always taken care of. How will they survive without us? Again so many questions without answers. My mother, who was diagnosed first and expected to die before her husband, began preparing frozen dinners so that when she was gone he would have food to eat. How will he live without me? Could he have been having the same thoughts? Were they powerful enough to end his life?

My stepfather, on the other hand, even in his denial, made sure his Living Trust was updated and his financial affairs in order so his children and grandchildren would be secure. Those actions say something about the actuality of his denial. Did he truly believe he was going to be cured or was it just a surface mechanism played out for us his survivors?

Living with a life threatening illness and the decline in capacity presents a series of losses; loss of identity, loss of control, of physical functions, of time, and of money.

We lose our sense of identity. We become a medical number, a patient in bed two. It seems when we trade our clothes for the backless hospital gown we also exchange our personhood for a disease.

Our identity is connected to who we perceive ourselves to be when we look in the mirror. I remember my mother crying in front of the bathroom mirror saying, "Who is that old woman looking back at me?" Here was a woman who was a professional model in her younger years, who took great pride in her appearance, watching her physical beauty slip away.

When we receive a diagnosis of any illness, it seems we give away the control of our well-being to strangers. The world of Marcus Welby is an example of a day gone by. Today HMOs and PPOs dictate the choice of our physician. From family practitioner to specialist, we are shifted from one stranger to another. Most often we do not know the qualifications of those we see. Were we referred to the Oncologist because he/she is the most qualified, or were we referred because they share the same clinic, medical group, or hospital affiliation? Or maybe the doctors are just golf buddies?

Because of this lack of control and the underlying insecurity about our care, we resort to idealization and rationalization about our physicians and care. "The Mayo Clinic said our doctors here were as fine as you could find anywhere." "Our doctor is the best Oncologist in the city". We always have the "best" doctor. Who else could we entrust with our life?

We are so vulnerable. In our fear and uncertainty, in our diminished physical and mental state, with our selective hearing and with our stress-induced emotions, we are making life-affecting decisions. We really need advocates to be with us, to help us see and hear clearly, to help us ask pertinent questions. The advocate should not necessarily be our spouse or close relative, since they are bringing as much baggage into any meeting as we are.

PHYSICAL FUNCTIONS

With any illness, we experience weakness and lack of energy but we also expect, as treatment begins to take affect, our energy to return. We expect that we will feel better. This is not so with the treatments associated with cancer. Instead of feeling better, we will probably start feeling worse. Our condition will continue to deteriorate. We begin living an oxymoron. We are receiving treatment yet feeling worse. We wonder, when will I ever feel better again?

As mentioned earlier, our mental clarity is also affected. We just don't have the energy to think. Don lamented one day that he didn't have the physical agility or energy to negotiate the stairs in the back yard to work on his roses, and he didn't have the mental clarity or focus to work on the book he was writing. All he could do was sit or sleep.

Imagine the embarrassment and humiliation an independent, macho, "one of the boys" kind of guy feels when he has to use a cane for balance. And then he has to have the cane replaced by a walker, and finally a wheelchair. No wonder he would disconnect his oxygen and wheel himself from the hos-

pital floor to the outside entrance and have a cigarette. What else did he have control of? What else
could he do?

The outside environment, the "normal" environment, is not made for the disabled. Oh, we talk about
it, we put up a few ramps and handlebars, but over-
all consciousness is not attuned to the challenged.

I took my mother to a shopping mall. She so enjoyed
shopping. To begin the adventure we had to get the
wheelchair into the trunk of the car, then get her, the
oxygen stroller and large purse (big enough to hold
all the pills, cough syrup bottle and atomizers) situ-
ated. Then it was off to the mall. We got out of the
car in the parking lot with as much effort as getting
into the car at home. Across the mall, the doors to
the entrance did not have an automatic opener, so
with agility I got the chair and myself inside before
it closed on my heels.

A department store is generally not geared for wheelchairs. The racks are so close together it is almost impossible to steer a wheelchair around. We basically were confined to the major aisles. Despite our handicaps, we made some major purchases--but that presented another obstacle. Where were we going to put everything when I needed my hands to push the chair? Mother, of course, held the sacks, but we also had a large box with which to contend. We put the box on the footrest with her feet on top of the box and to the car we went, laughing all the way. What is the saying about making lemonade?

LOSS OF TIME

Time is the enemy, for the patient and for the care-giver. There just isn't enough of it. It speeds by so quickly; a day is gone, a week is gone, a month is gone, a life is gone. So much time wasted. So much centered on the illness and not enough on living. So little spent in joy.

For the patient the issue is lack of energy. "Maybe I will feel better tomorrow." A rule of thumb is to assume each day is as good as it is going to get and live accordingly. Live each day to the best that the body and mind will allow.

The caregiver has other issues to contend with and adjust to. Most of us had a very full and often stressful life before our loved one became ill. Our days were packed then. Now we probably still have all the original activities with the addition of caring for someone who progressively needs help in all areas of their life.

There aren't enough hours in the day to accomplish all that we need to do. There are doctor's appointments, lab visits, medications to pick up, maybe home health or hospice visits to be present for, plus the physical care; giving of medicines, maybe assisting with dressing and bathing. All of this in addition to cooking, cleaning, the everyday "normal" routines.

I got a new insight into hospice and home health visits being on the other side of hospice when my mother was receiving care in my home. I certainly looked forward to the visits of the RN, social worker, volunteer and the home health aide. The reassurance of the nurse's perspective was my security blanket. The listening ear of the social worker was my sounding board. The bathing and bed change by the home health aide gave me extra minutes to myself for quiet time or to do something that needed to be done that I just hadn't found the time to do.

In spite of all the value I gained from each and every visit, it was a disruption. I had to be "on" for someone entering my home. I had to put what I was doing on hold until the visit was over. It was one more time-stealing event. From this experience, as a health care professional, I learned to say what needs to be said and do whatever is appropriate for the visit in a non-rushed manner, but quickly and time efficiently.

The home health aide time frame is too individualized to give an estimate. For a hospice nurse or social worker visit, just about everything can be accomplished between 45 and 90 minutes. Anything over that generally, and there are always exceptions, was too much talk and a waste. Don't stay too long. It is a theft of time.

LOSS OF MONEY AND TIME FOR MEDICAL EXPENSES

Each day, when both of my parents were still in their home but ill, the mail would bring several envelopes containing medical statements; some insurance, some Medicare. They were supposed to understand the meaning of all of the forms and computer printouts. Some were asking for payment, some were requiring completion for reimbursement, all of them were complicated.

Here were two elderly people from a generation that is extremely conscientious about paying their bills in a timely manner. They were both sick, therefore experiencing lack of energy and mental clarity, trying to figure out what to pay and what to expect to receive. They were frustrated and humiliated by their inability to complete a task that a short while ago they could have done.

INTERACTION WITH MEDICAL PROFESSIONALS

It was interesting to watch the social masks go on when encountering anyone outside of the family. Both of my parents had a change of personality for medical personnel.

Don may have been in pain and frightened, but for the family he was the protector, for the lab personnel he was the stoic, for the female nurses and aides he was the gentleman, and for the male doctors he was one of the guys. He was never the vulnerable, sick, frightened man that lived inside of his body. He talked football and music systems with his doctors but not the personal progress of his body. Sadly, the doctors played his game.

My mother, on the other hand, was the coquette, the cute little girl with the male doctors and the passive, "I'm sick but no problems" woman with the rest of the medical professionals. I remember her complaining at length about her swallowing. I suggested we talk with the hospice nurse about it. During the visit I was waiting for her to bring the subject up for discussion. Finally I said, "Did you forget to tell Jean about your swallowing?" "Oh, that is nothing" she said but Jean took over from there and the issue was addressed.

It is so important that we as health care professionals speak in a language that is understandable. I took Dorothy to a doctor's appointment. As the doctor was explaining her condition, she sat on the examining table nodding her head in agreement and understanding. But I, a hospice nurse, did not understand the terminology and phraseology he was using so I knew she didn't.

I think, depending on the personality type, it can all be so overwhelming. So much to hear, to remember, to understand. We feel small in the room, there without our clothes, so vulnerable. If we say we don't understand, that we may never understand, we will feel even smaller. We are scared, overwhelmed and don't have the energy or clarity to comprehend. We need an advocate, someone we can believe and trust.

Everything is moving so fast; it's all a blur. Health care professionals need to slow the pace, speak clearly and distinctly, using non-medical terminology. They need to sit down, use bonding skills, be honest and direct yet gentle. They can help their patients and families make decisions based on true facts, on real options, by recognizing the impaired position in which illness puts a person.

Generally every word uttered by a medical professional is golden. Words are retained and made concrete when the person saying them is not even aware they have said them. I'm sure the doctor did not mean anything serious when he suggested to a patient of mine to "watch your sugar intake," but she stopped eating all sugar. The Oncologist, at the beginning of her diagnosis, told my mother if she didn't have radiation she would be dead in six months (not a very tactful bedside manner, by the way). Because she did not have radiation, she became convinced she would die in November, six months from the time of his pronouncement. In December, she finally admitted I might have been right about her not dying at that time. She lived another year and three months from that November.

Professionals need to be so careful of what is said. Not only for what is actually said, but what is implied. They need to verify what the patient and family are really hearing as well as check for how much they are retaining.

HOSPICE

As a hospice nurse, I thought I could convince anyone of the benefits of becoming a hospice patient. If they had a limited prognosis, then they needed hospice concepts and philosophy to help them with this part of their life experience. Hospice could certainly make a difference in a person's quality of life. I believed in what I "preached" and I was good at "selling" hospice—until I had to talk to my own parents.

Don did not accept hospice as an option because he was, after all, going to "beat this thing." His doctors supported him in his decision. To them, hospice was a conflict of interest in their approach to cure.

Dorothy was a different matter. She was receptive to any of my suggestions regarding her care. She had tremendous trust and faith in my knowledge. I was in one city and she three hundred miles away in another. I wanted a hospice there to begin assisting her. I thought I would then have a reliable source of information on her status and she would have the support that I couldn't give her from a distance.

The difficulty came when I began talking about hospice and how it would help both of us. Her shocked response was I must think she was going to die-now.

Hospice has a bad public relations image. The message the public is given is that hospice takes care of people who are dying. Because of this, people are reluctant to even think about hospice care, let alone sign the papers. If I sign the papers, then I know and acknowledge that I will be dead in six months. This is so frightening.

What generally happens is the person who is sick has actually begun the labor of dying and it is the family that accepts the hospice help. Now the person looks like death is near so hospice is recognized as timely.

In reality, hospice does a wonderful job of helping people live the best they can within the confines that their disease and body has put them in. When the referral comes weeks or days before death, it can really only provide crisis intervention.

So back to mother. We talked at length about how hospice could help us, that no one knows how long a person has to live, but we do know she can't be fixed and the disease will just keep growing. Hospice helps people who can't be fixed to live better.

We called a local hospice, and while I was in town they did an assessment visit and the Medicare papers were signed. Service began after I left to return home. No home health aide was provided because mother was too independent. Oxygen was supplied, but no oxygen stroller. It was not their policy. The social worker never did show up. Medicare would not have approved of that. There was no talk of volunteers. A nurse showed up once a week, took vital signs, and left. Mother's cough syrup was paid for.

You know the saying, "A rose is a rose is a rose."

Well, a hospice is a hospice is not a hospice! What my mother was receiving was home health care billed as hospice care with the cough syrup paid for.

Where was the bonding, the support, the listening? There wasn't any. I came again to visit and called to talk with the nurse. I called the office three times in a forty-five minute period beginning at 10 a.m. I got no response from the nurse and no one else offered to assist us. At 4 p.m. the nurse called and gave me her excuse for not returning my call. I don't even remember what the excuse was now, it was unimportant. What was important is my mother and I put our lives on hold for six hours--six hours we did not have to waste, because of someone else's lack of consideration. This was not hospice care. Hospice knows better!

Following Don's death in September, I brought Dorothy to live with me and we transferred to a hospice near me. The difference in hospices was striking. Mother arrived coughing, complaining of a sore mouth and not eating. She was very tired and depressed and sick, and I thought she would be dead before Thanksgiving.

The hospice nurse arrived for the initial assessment. Following the get acquainted, gathering information period, she began offering her suggestions. She wanted to change cough syrups to a suppressant instead of an expectorant. She tested for Thrush, recommended she talk to the doctor about a small dosage of Prednisone to increase appetite, and possibly an antidepressant. The social worker was scheduled for several times a week to listen and help us process not only mother's own end of life issues, but also the recent death of her husband and my step-father. Volunteers would be weekly visitors to give me, the caregiver, an opportunity to leave the house. As importantly, the volunteers would bring friendship to Dorothy since she knew no one other than her family.

Within a week, mother was new person. The strangling coughing was gone. She was eating better. She had more energy and although, naturally sad at her circumstances, was able to enjoy day-to-day happenings.

A hospice is a hospice is NOT a hospice. There is an expertise to end of life care. It is a specialty area. Being Medicare certified as a hospice does not guarantee expertise.

As I reread the above paragraphs, my thought was, "If you know enough to write this book, then why on earth didn't you recognize these needs in your own mother?" What is the saying, "A lawyer that has himself for a client has a fool for a lawyer?" When someone we care about has a problem, all objectivity goes out the window. We become so immersed in our own feelings, fears and concerns that our area of expertise is clouded. An important thing I told both hospices was that I may be a hospice professional, but I was Dorothy's daughter first. I thought, felt and reacted as a daughter, not as a nurse or hospice director.

I remember standing in the hall asking the hospice nurse how long she thought mother had to live. How many times had I lectured about families always asking just that question and how many times had I given the answer Jean gave to me? The difference was now I was the caregiver and all I could feel was exhaustion.

ASSISTANCE

Bathing is an American ritual. We take our baths seriously and very frequently. Having to not only maintain one's own personal hygiene but also assist another with theirs can become cumbersome and very time consuming. I didn't comprehend the magnitude of something as simple as bathing until I had to fit assisting with one into my day.

Colleen began helping Dorothy with her shower three days a week as soon as hospice services began. Oh what help it was to have that free forty-five minutes to an hour while she helped with a morning routine and changed the bed. Mother had found a new friend and grew to care for Colleen deeply. They visited, laughed and cried together. Colleen was a healing presence for both of us.

The visits of the three women--nurse, social worker and aide--became focal points of each week. We looked forward to their time with us, but we also had the rest of the week to live through. It was important to know the scheduling of these visits. We were establishing a routine, and like any good routine, it depended on timeliness. It was very important to us to know when each person was going to arrive. Setting an approximate time on a given day helped us plan the rest of our day. Calling at the beginning of the day to confirm the visit gave us a sense of security in our very insecure world.

It is wise to not give a specific time of arrival but give an approximate time. If you tell me you are coming at 9 a.m. and arrive at 9:15 you are late. If you tell me you are coming sometime between 9:00 and 10:00 and arrive at 9:15, then you show me you can be trusted.

Follow-through is so important in establishing a relationship. If a health care professional says they are going to do something, no matter how small, then I, as a patient or caregiver, believe them. I look to you as the expert, as my savior in an environment in which I feel very helpless. Don't let me down by not following through. I need to be able to trust what you say. If I can rely on you in small things, I can probably rely on you in the areas where I feel the most lost.

Trust and bonding is a major factor in a hospice relationship. As a patient and a caregiver, we look to the professional for guidance. We are overwhelmed, tired, vulnerable and very frightened. Fear walks with us all the time. Hospice becomes our saving grace. Hospice will provide the answers. Hospice will be there when we feel alone. Hospice will comfort us.

Our world is filled with so many strangers that we are forced to depend upon. We are looking for a point of stability, and that stability becomes the hospice care team. We are like baby ducks fresh out of the shell, and the first people we see from hospice become our Light. We will follow them anywhere if given the warmth and humanness we so desperately need.

CAREGIVER

As open and direct as my relationship was with my mother, there were still things I didn't want to talk about in front of her. The nurse may have called on a day when I wanted to strangle my mother, but when Jean said, "How are you," with mother sitting at the table by the phone, I only felt comfortable saying, "fine." If Jean had said, "can you talk now?" I would have been able to set up another time when we could talk more freely.

There was also tension when I would walk the nurse or social worker to the car and visit in the driveway. Upon my return to the house I was generally met with, "Were you talking about me?"

There is no perfect relationship; it is never all

smooth and wonderful. I left home when I was eighteen and did quite well in the ensuing forty-two years without maternal guidance, yet when Mother moved in our relationship regressed to one of a mother and an eighteen year old. It took some intervention and guidance on the part of the social worker to help us get our roles straight.

Mother and I were encouraged to see each other for the women we were now, and to acknowledge the unique situation today presented us. We were given the opportunity to "get it right" with each other. If we could let go of the past and concentrate on each day together, we had the chance of creating some special time now that we could share.

In order to work on our relationship, it was I who had to change. Mother was just too sick. Her energy was decreasing. She did not have the stamina to work on issues. By my changing, she responded to me in a different manner and our relationship blossomed.

First, I let go of what I wanted from her. The little girl in me stopped trying to get the attention and love from a mother who gave the most she had. The fact that it didn't seem enough to me was my issue, not hers. The social worker said, "Love is a verb." It is an action word. I was showing my love in my caring. I learned to love the woman in front of me each day for what she was that day. I set boundaries, but I gave unconditional love.

In response, my mother became open, funny, sweet, a beautiful person to be with. In the last four months of her life, we had all the facets of the relationship I had always wanted. By giving, I received more than I had ever imagined.

QUALITY TIME

Once mother was first diagnosed and the shock began to wear off, one of my first thoughts was how do we make what time there is left special? How do we begin building memories?

Holidays are always memory-builders, but now they were bittersweet. The underlying thought of everyone was that each holiday gathering would probably be our last with her. And true to course, there was a last of each--but how fortunate we all were to at least know there was a last one. We took the gift of time that was offered. We did not waste it.

Now, with hindsight, I remember most the afternoon at Glamour Shots where the girls in the family all laughed, tried on clothes and posed. Mother, at 76 flirted with the photographer and did her modeling thing.

Also a standout in my mind is the two-week trip across country to see my son's play with six people living in an RV. Be careful of the memories you build--an RV gets crowded with six people 24/7.

We took a lot of pictures. People tend to not take pictures of those who are ill. They certainly are not looking their best, but work with what you have because the photos are the preservation of memories. The picture of a woman who didn't care for cats, asleep in a hospital bed, with five cats asleep in various positions around her brings smiles and initiates memories.

The memories built during a time of approaching death can be the kind you savor or the kind that make you cringe. The choice is up to us as participants in the end of life experience.

Our choice was to find the joy in each day. When I

would tuck Dorothy in at night, I would sit on the side of her bed and ask her what was good about the day. I would listen as she would recount the day. Sometimes it was simply watching television together or sharing a candy bar. One day she couldn't find anything good and we talked about how we let that happen.

We learned that everyone needs a purpose for getting up in the morning. In the months before death, when the person is still eating, has energy and an interest in activity, a sense of purpose is at its lowest. They get up, get dressed, but then what? Aimlessness sets in. There really isn't enough energy to physically do what you could once do. It is a challenge to find daily activities that promote interest and self-worth. As energy decreases and withdrawal begins, purpose becomes less of an issue.

An activity we found valuable was to record a family history. Dorothy tape-recorded her memories of her family. This was an opportunity for her to do a life review while helping us preserve our heritage. In the early months she also, with the help of the hospice volunteers, created a hook rug for her soon to be born great-grandchild, and she wrote her children letters to be read when she was gone. She had purpose while she needed it.

Don died in the hospital. The cancerous tumor had shrunk, but the radiation had so scarred his lungs that he died of respiratory failure, a side effect of radiation. I had driven in to take him to his home, the doctors finally admitting there was nothing more they could do. I spent the night in the hospital room sleeping on a cot beside his bed. Don and I finally had an in-depth, "this is the situation" talk at his initiation. I was always ready to talk, which he knew; our agreement had been when he was ready, he would ask. As part of our conversation, I told him there was nothing more that could be done for him. We would take him home and keep him comfortable. He said he wanted to do just that. After the talk, I literally watched the tension leave him.

During the night he would open his eyes, turn his head to look at me, smile then close his eyes. At some point during the night he entered a deep sleep, eyes partially open, and became non-responsive. Labor had begun.

We, as a family, stayed with him during the following day. We acknowledged that there was no need to take him home, death was too close for a transfer.

As evening came, Mother and I said our goodbyes and left for home. Mother was too sick herself for a night vigil. My sister and her daughter stayed with Don. He died gently during the night with his daughter and granddaughter at his side.

We die the way we have lived and according to our personality. Don was closest to my sister and her daughter. He was protective of his wife and knew I would be her protector in his absence. His coping mechanism was to deny and fight. When there was nothing more to fight for, he died. He had a labor of 24 hours. He was a doer personality. A long labor was not his approach to life.

Dorothy died in my living room. She waited for her other daughter and granddaughter to arrive from out of state. We were all sitting in the kitchen sharing stories, her bed just on the other side of the wall, when my daughter heard a sound. She went into the room as mother took her last breath.

Her family was close. We had all said our goodbyes. My daughter had told her grandmother she wanted to be with her when she left this world. She was. Mother died the way she had lived. Independent, but with family close.

Following the funeral, my daughter, who had helped her grandmother write letters to her daughters by writing as she dictated her thoughts, passed on this letter. Her simple words gave confirmation to the journey we had experienced together.

My Dearest Barbara,
There aren't words to say how I feel about you. We have worked together to make this go as long as we could. It's coming to an end and only God can take the last breath from me.
I'll miss (our time) in the office and evenings in the family room, the laughing, the dinners, the joys of life.
I get joy out of being with you.
The many, many hours we have never been together to get to know each other and now we have come to our goal.
We have learned how we feel about each other.
There was never time to get close before but now we have come together in a sad and happy way.
We have to part, but it is not my choice. It was fun

while it lasted.
Every night I'll miss those hugs and kisses.
I love you very much!
PS. I'll be down to give you hugs and kisses too.

Living with a life threatening illness and experiencing the inevitable death, although frightening and certainly challenging, is a gift of opportunity. It is the opportunity to make it "right" with the relationship, to address any unfinished business, to live in the present and to say goodbye. It is a blessing, not the curse as seen by so many.

GRIEF

MALE VERSES FEMALE

VISITATION AND FUNERAL

CREMATION

CHILDREN

NOTES:

This chapter is obviously not everything that was ever written about grief. It is only about normal grieving, the process that occurs when we suffer a loss. That loss can be termed a death. There are many kinds of deaths, death of a marriage, death of a relationship, death of a lifestyle, death from a change of location, death of a job and what we most associate as a death, the death of a physical body.

Imagine a long table sitting in front of an open window. On the table are tidy stacks of papers. A gentle breeze comes through the open window and ruffles the papers; they stay in their stacks, but barely. Now a big gust of wind sends the papers flying all over the room. Grieving is like this. Most of the time we have our emotions in a tidy arrangement, under control and manageable. But there are days when we wake up and just under the surface the feelings of our loss are stirring. We have control, almost. It is like "if someone looks at me funny I may cry; if someone doesn't look at me funny I may cry." Then there are days we wake up and start crying before our feet hit the floor. That is the day we call in sick, stay home, go through the photo albums, feel very sorry for ourselves and cry all day. Our emotions are scattered all over the place.

Grief is a whole group of emotions wrapped into one package we call grieving and mourning but it also manifests in our body as actual physical pain. There is a knot or clinching in the stomach area; our heart is screaming; we are restless and anxious or experience fatigue, we sleep too much or can't sleep enough. We physically feel our grief.

Grief is the emotion of loneliness. "I am so lonely. I am all alone now." This loneliness is two fold. It is self-imposed, but it also comes from the absence of a support network.

We tend to isolate ourselves when our grieving begins. We just don't have the energy to do anything. Sometimes it is too much to just get dressed. We can't seem to focus. We are numb. We just go through the motions of being alive.

Being with others is helpful and distracting but others tend to be uncomfortable around us. We don't have the inclination to reach out to others, and others seem to avoid us. There is often awkwardness in people about not knowing what to say to us. Others can see us, we appear "stable," not crying, functioning, so they are afraid to really ask us how we are, to even bring up the subject of our loss for fear we may react and they won't know what to do. So they stay away and we are lonely.

What people need to know is that our deceased loved one is in our mind all the time in early grief. A second doesn't go by that we don't miss them. We are learning how to go on living minute by minute. By you talking directly and openly about our loved one, you allow us to verbalize memories and feelings. It helps. Yes, we may cry, but that is okay. It helps the loneliness to talk. Share your memories of the person that is gone, use their name, help us know they touched your life, that they are missed by you also.

Grief is, "I'm sad. I am so sad that he is no longer in my life. I miss him so much." The sadness is a feeling deep within us that resonates no matter what we are doing. It is so intense it can almost be physically located within our body.

Grief also manifests in feelings of anger. "I am so angry!" We are angry at the changes that have been forced upon us. Changes we didn't request out of life. Changes that have made us unhappy and sad. Our life, because of a death, has incurred complications for which we were not prepared. There are new responsibilities, often financial concerns as the result of medical bills and loss of income. We may now be a single parent with all the trials that come with raising children alone. All of these changes are because someone prominent in our life died. We become frustrated and mad. Mad at the person who died and left us with these challenges. Mad at God for letting this happen. Mad at the doctors and nurses for not doing their job. And mad at ourselves--for what, we are not sure.

When we are angry with ourselves, we tend not to share these feelings with others. We feel guilty about having all these angry thoughts and often think if anyone were to know what we are thinking and feeling they would think less of us, so we hold those feelings in and become depressed.

Grief is, "I am so depressed." Anger held inward

becomes depression. Depression by itself, without a loss, has all the signs of normal grieving; lack of appetite, difficulty sleeping (or the opposite over-sleeping), isolation, numbness, apathy, confusion, crying. People can be depressed and not grieving, but generally people who are grieving are depressed.

Grief is, "I am frightened." We think about all the things we were told to do during the illness, of all the things we did to stay healthy and live a "good" life. We ate the correct foods, we exercised. We took the treatments but our special person died anyway and that means we could die too.

Death of someone close to us makes us face our own mortality and the mortality of those around us. We begin to worry more about being in cars, about the welfare of our children, of ourselves. Death shows us how little control over our lives we really have. It destroys the illusion that we will live forever. It is frightening to feel like a ship adrift in the sea of life. Our rudder, our stabilizer in life, is generally the belief that if we do what is "right" we will survive. Now we have questions of "What is right?", "Does it really matter?", and "Where do I go from here?" It is scary to have our beliefs shaken.

Grief is, "I am lonely, I am sad, I am angry, I am depressed, I am frightened, and I don't seem to be in control." As you can see, grief centers around us, the "I", not really around the person that has died. It is very self-centered. I have gotten criticism for approaching grief in this manner, but I don't mean self-centered in a negative way.

Our Judeo-Christian belief teaches us that when we are dead we are in a better place--that living is hard work and being dead is easy. With that belief in mind, then the person who is dead is better off than we are. We are the ones who have to deal with the guilt, the questions without answers, and the difficult task of building a life from an empty space. Our grief is about us, how we feel, how we react, how we cope.

Unfortunately, in our society, because we tend to not identify with the self-centeredness of grieving, we look for solutions outside of ourselves instead of looking within. Our life situation is forcing us to change and that is very difficult. No one can make those adjustments for us. It is our show all the way.

All of these feelings are normal and natural. They are part of the normal grieving process. They are going to be a part of our life for a while. We should allow ourselves to feel them. To often, because actually feeling all of these emotions and accepting them hurts too much, we run from them. We keep ourselves very busy. Run, run, run, the busier we are the less we have time to experience how awful we really feel. Once we stop and acknowledge our feelings and accept them, we can begin to learn how to go on living.

If I cut my arm, a deep gash clear to the bone, I would have to go to the emergency center. They would anesthetize the area and stitch the wound. It would heal from the inside out and form a scar. I have a scar on my leg that I got when I was twelve years old; at sixty, when I touch the scar it still feels different from the rest of my body.

Grief is like that wound. The depth of the cut relates to the depth of our emotional relationship with the person who has died. A child or spouse's death is the deepest cut of all.

There is no greater loss than the death of a child. Our children are our legacy to the world. It must be written somewhere in the law of life that parents die before their children. When our children die that law is broken. A major piece of ourself dies.

To continue the wound analogy let's say a spouse has died. Our wound is immense. At first we are numb, we are on automatic pilot. We get through the visitation and the funeral. We do and say all the right things. We cry, we hurt, but basically we are numb.

Then six weeks, three months later, we fall in a little heap on the floor. We begin to think there is something seriously wrong with us mentally. We must be going crazy because we are more emotional and less stable than we were at the funeral.

What has happened is the anesthetic that Life has given us for the wound has worn off. Now we feel the real pain of grieving. The church ladies are no longer bringing over the tuna casserole; the kids are not calling every night. Everyone has returned to their normal lives and activities and we realize nothing is "normal" for us anymore. We have to begin building a new life, a life without our special person.

At first our loved one is in our mind every moment. Not a waking minute goes by that we aren't missing them, and we hope when we are able to sleep we will dream of them to feel their closeness. As time goes by we venture out, have lunch with friends and return to our empty home to realize we didn't think of our missed one all afternoon. Then a day out brings all day without thinking of them.

A frightening time comes when we can't pull their face into our mind's eye and we have to get out the scrapbook to see them clearly.

Then one day we are walking down the grocery aisle and stop in front of the oatmeal section and begin crying. We remember that our loved one ate oatmeal every day and how much we miss them. We didn't get to tell them about our life's events, about the kids, about the world. We miss them so much and it has been ten years since they have died. A memory touched the scar and we felt the pain all over again.

I think at some point (and the timing is different for everyone) we decide to put our active grief behind us and move forward. For some of us, it is a conscious moment. Others, without even realizing it, move back into the stream of life. In hindsight, most of us can identify that time in our grieving when we began building a new life.

Even with building a new life, grief doesn't go away. We don't heal or even recover from grief. We have to learn how to live with it. There are no words or pills that can take our grief away and make us feel better. Only time affects grief. Time extends the space between the memories and the pain.

We will never be the same again. There is no going back to what we had before the death. Yes, we dream about going back, want to go back, to recapture what we had, but it is gone. The past becomes a loss also.

There is no time frame on grieving. Many factors influence the effect the loss will have on us. Grieving is as individual and as unique as is each human being. The nature of our relationship to the deceased will affect the gravity of our grief. The intensity of our emotional involvement is equal to the intensity of our grief. That involvement can be a negative relationship as well as a positive one. I can be overwhelmed with grief for a divorced spouse that I have unresolved feeling about. I can grieve less for the blood cousin that I had no relationship with except for holidays.

Unfinished business, a dysfunctional relationship and the need for closure also affects the length of grieving. These areas often lead to pathological grieving and the need for professional bereavement counseling.

There is no magic 366th-day when we move forward in our grief experience. Some say the second year is actually harder than the first.

During the first year our friends and family are generally supportive. Everyone is attuned to the first Christmas, the first Thanksgiving, the first birthday, the first anniversary, and the death day. By the second year, those not as close to our loss have resumed their lives, filled in the empty space and are wondering why we haven't. It is not necessarily uncaring on their part as much as ignorance to the depth of the void we have to fill. There just isn't as much support in the second year and we find ourselves still lonely, sad, angry and depressed; still grieving, just not as intensely. Time indeed is beginning to fill in the space death leaves.

MALE GRIEF VS. FEMALE GRIEF

Men and women experience the same emotions of grieving. If grief is defined as loneliness, sadness, anger, fear, depression--as well as physical manifestations due to a loss--then men and women grieve in the same way. The expression of that grief is different, however.

Picture a get-together for a women's bridge club. I arrive and tearfully say I am having a difficult day. I verbalize my feelings of sadness. There will probably be seven other women that will nurture and support me that afternoon. A lot of bridge may not get played, but I will be listened to. I have a hard time picturing that same scenario at a men's poker game.

Because men are generally not expressive with their emotions, they do not get the support they need to be comforted. Their persona says, "I am fine," when in reality they are not.

There seems to be a time line, a generation identity, involving emotionality in men. Men sixty and over have a more difficult time with their emotions than men under sixty. I am making generalities here; there are of course exceptions. Society taught men over sixty to be macho, in charge, in control, and said that tears were a sign of weakness. "Big boys don't cry" was how they were raised, so they learned to suppress their feelings. As a culture we are doing better with this myth, but it is still in evidence to some extent.

Grief, when not expressed outwardly, often comes forth physically as illness. The mortality rate of widowers in the first year of grief is much higher than widows. This can be directly attributed to men not figuring out how to go on living.

The partnership of marriage, particularly in the older generation, is one where the wife is generally not only the cook and dish washer but very often also the banker, business manger, and social arranger as well as best friend and confidant. When that wife dies, there is a tremendous void.

I remember sitting at a kitchen table with a gentle-man in his seventies while we were waiting for the funeral home workers to arrive to take his wife's body to the mortuary. As he was appropriately crying, he said he just didn't know how he was going to live without her. He explained he didn't know how to cook, how to do the laundry, or how much money was in the bank. He was totally unprepared to live on his own.

Unfortunately, this gentleman's situation is not unique. Many of our senior men do not have the skills for single living. This adds an additional stressor to their grieving, and additional tasks of learning how to go on living.

One of the solutions to lack of single living skills is to remarry. Very often within six months to a year the widower will find a new wife.

Our community and families often do not respond favorably or supportively when the newly widowed remarry. This lack of support is sad and very unfortunate. We let some myths and biases get in the way of our compassion. Adult children often respond negatively with, "Dad didn't really love Mom if he can marry this 'gold digger' now," "50 years of marriage and it was all a sham," "What in the world is Dad thinking of? In his grief has he become mentally ill, or does he have dementia?"

Adult children need to be helped to find a different, more understanding perspective. In their own grief they are failing to see that love doesn't end with death or with remarriage. There are many kinds of love and as many reasons for it. We can truly love more than one person at a time. Parenthood is proof of that. To marry another does not take away from a life of caring and love for one that is no longer with us.

I am not suggesting that remarriage is the answer to a grieving husband with no survival skills or for a man who is lonely and wants companionship. That road chosen will be very difficult indeed. The person is still in active grieving and is really not himself yet. A challenge for the new wife is that there are only saints in cemeteries and it is very difficult to live with the memory of a recently departed wife.

Unfortunately, most people upon their deaths are

immediately elevated into sainthood. We promptly forget all their humanness and imperfections, and they become the most wonderful person that ever lived. Their perfections give us the reason for our pain and feelings of great loss. By selective remembering we can build a fantasy past to comfort us in our uncertain future. Of course, it is more constructive to try to keep a memory balanced, to keep in perspective that no person is all good or all bad. Life and its experiences, along with all of us humans, is imperfect.

VISITATION AND FUNERAL

I was taking care of a family when the primary care giver died before the patient. This was a multigenerational family living in one home, a thirty year-old woman, her mother and father, in their late fifties, and the grandmother in her eighties. The grandmother was the hospice patient and her daughter was the primary care giver. The fifty year old daughter just dropped dead one day. I attended the visitation to pay my respects to the family. As I entered the funeral home, the remaining family were seated in the front row of the viewing room; I walked over and visited for a few moments with each person and then walked to the casket to say my goodbyes to the body. People walked about or gathered in groups, but the family remained seated in the front row.

Several weeks later, the grandmother died and I was again at the same funeral home attending a visitation. Again the immediate family was seated in the front row of the viewing room. I visited with the family while they sat and then walked to the casket to say my goodbyes. I returned to the family and as I was talking the adult daughter commented on how much she would like to get up and have a cigarette. I suggested that she do that, but she said the funeral director had told them when her mother died that they were to sit in the front row during the visitation.

She believed she couldn't leave her seat until everyone had gone.

This family had never been involved in a funeral or visitation service before. They did not know how to do it. They took the funeral director's suggestion literally as to how a visitation was conducted. They did not know they could walk around, visit or smoke. They didn't have a role model from which to draw.

From that experience I learned not to assume people know they can have any kind of a service they want; that they can bury their loved one in pajamas or baseball uniforms; that they can play favorite music, display pictures and tell stories. Part of my teaching to families is about visitation and funeral options.

Visitations and funerals are really for the living, not the dead. Their function is to bring family and friends together to celebrate the life of the one who has gone before us. Visitations are called visitations because we visit with and find support in those gathered around us.

Viewing the body is not the focal point of a visitation, but it is a very healthful part. In today's society we are conducting more and more memorial services and fewer visitations of the body and funerals with the coffin present. We want to avoid discomfort so we have a service without the coffin, generally with a nice picture of the deceased instead. As painful as it is to see someone we care about laid out in a casket, it leaves no doubt in our mind that death has occurred. Until we understand, experience and encounter the actual pain of loss, our grieving is incomplete. An open casket facilitates the grieving process.

The expense of a visitation and funeral does not say

how much we love or care about the person that has died, yet we often get confused about this and spend way too much money. We can create meaning to the events without spending a great deal. A blanket of roses to cover the coffin is beautiful, but costly. When my stepfather died we purchased a red rose from each member of the family, a white rose to represent my mother, and a tiny pink rosebud to symbolize my niece's unborn child. Those roses with baby's breath and a banner saying, "We love you," were laid upon the casket. Those flowers had more meaning for us than any other bouquet of flowers could. They cost $75.00. We later dried the flowers and had them made into a wreath, which we placed upon the headstone.

Visitations and funerals are for our comfort. There are many creative ways to find that comfort. As the family gathers before the service, talk can be about what will be meaningful and helpful. My sister's husband made a tape of my stepfather's favorite music, which was played during the visitation. The cassette was then placed in my stepfather's pocket as a "going away" present.

Generally there is a receiving line where the family stands to the side of the coffin to meet with and acknowledge the friends who are paying their respects. The guests move to the casket for viewing and then move on. Having an easel or table with a collage of pictures of the deceased on the other side of the casket, opposite the receiving line, is an excellent way of celebrating the life that has ended.

Family photos, wedding pictures, and vacation pictures become the gathering spot for people as they remember and reminisce about a life lived.

Gathering the pictures is a good family project, which helps in grieving and mourning. It brings people together with a purpose. It encourages memory sharing and story telling. It also helps celebrate the life.

During the time following the death and before the visitation, I recommend that each significant person in the life of the deceased write an actual letter to the person who has died; to put down on paper all that is in their hearts. Because life is neither all good nor all bad, because there are happy and sad times to every relationship, address all the feelings that need to be expressed. The letter can be a note simply saying, "I love you and will miss you," or it can be many pages covering a lifetime of thoughts and emotions. No one needs to see what is written. This need not be shared with anyone. Quietly place it somewhere in the coffin during the private viewing.

Children can draw pictures and/or place their school picture with their letter. Again, be creative. I have had bodies covered with pictures and letters. I have had letters discreetly placed underneath the hands, in pockets and under pillows. It is all individual and comforting. There is something very powerful about having to focus our thoughts into words and make them concrete by putting them on paper. It is okay to talk to our loved one and tell them what is in our hearts, but writing to them is very healing.

In writing a letter to someone that has died, it doesn't have to be immediate and placed in the coffin. If someone has died and you still have something you need to say to them, positive or negative, even if it has been twenty years since their death--write them a letter. Write whatever you need to say to have closure and then do something special with the letter. Burn it and scatter the ashes, or put the letter in a special place or container. It is a personal letter and does not have to be shared. It is our own private closure.

CREMATION

When there is cremation of the body there is usually a memorial service and most generally no viewing of the body. As I mentioned earlier, viewing of the body is an important step in grieving. That step does not have to be eliminated just because the choice is cremation. We can talk with the funeral director about a private viewing. It is also important to go ahead and spend the money for the cosmetics to be done on the body as well as dressing the body in our favorite clothes. Often mortuaries have a "rent a casket" type of program for the few minutes it takes to say our last goodbyes. Even if we were at the bedside when our special person died, it is not the same as standing looking into the casket and seeing the body prepared in death. This is the time we not only say our goodbyes but also place our carefully written letters, pictures or notes with the body. Here we can find closure.

When we close our eyes, we need a place to see our loved one resting. Cemeteries provide that place of comfort. If the ashes are scattered following cremation we do not have any place to go in our mind, or for that matter any place to go physically to feel we are close to the person we miss so much. There can be peace sitting by the gravesite.

I was hiking in the Oregon Mountains one time and came upon a beautiful waterfall. It was far removed from activity, towns and people, a lovely spot of unspoiled nature. There beside the stream was a white wooden cross with a wooden scroll attached to the cross bar. The scroll told the story of a young man's love of nature and his ashes being scattered in a place he felt at peace.

We need to find a special place that the memory of its location and purpose will bring comfort and peace to our being. Dropping ashes from an airplane or throwing ashes from a moving boat is generally too abstract for our mind to return to. A flower garden, an arboretum, a small lake, a mountain stream, an inlet are all areas that can be physically returned to in seeking closeness with our special person. Cemeteries now have gardens and beautiful areas where ashes can be kept.

CHILDREN AND GRIEF

I was fourteen when my grandfather died, a freshman in high school. My mother had not even told me he was sick, let alone that he was going to die. I was getting ready for school one morning and she said very matter of factly, "Grandpa died last night. I'm going to help Nana today while you are in school." Off to school I went. That night, when I was asking for details, I was told there would be a funeral but I could not attend because I "wasn't old enough." With all the insistence a fourteen year old is capable of, I argued that I wanted to go to the funeral. I didn't win the argument, but as a compromise I was taken to the funeral home to see Grandpa.

Without advance notice we arrived at the funeral home and were directed to a small upstairs room. The mortuary was an old Victorian house with many rooms, a grand wide central staircase and a narrow back staircase. We were directed to the narrow back staircase. I remember vividly the small candle-like wall sconces dimly lighting the stairs as we quietly ascended into a dark hall. At the top of the stairs we entered a room lit only by a glass covered candle placed at the head of the casket. There, in the coffin, was my grandfather. At that moment I knew with all my being that my mother had been right. If this was okay for me to see, and it was frightening me terribly, then a funeral was certainly something I was convinced I would never attend.

In my mother's efforts to protect me from a sad, uncomfortable experience, she had frightened me beyond words. I did not go to a funeral until I was in my mid-thirties and then I wouldn't view the body.

In an effort to protect our children, we often do more damage than good. Imagination is generally far worse than reality. We need to be open, honest, direct yet gentle with our children in preparing them for death and the rituals following death. Our goal is to help them understand the normalcy of death. Everybody dies. It is sad but it is not pathological. It is normal. It is confusing. It often doesn't seem right or "fair," but it happens. And when it does, we deal with it.

Death is a part of life, and by excluding our children from experiencing our involvement with dying and death, we are robbing them of the opportunity to learn an important segment of life. We are depriving them of the ability to learn how to cope with death. We are not giving them role models from which to build their life skills.

Too often we, as adults, pass on to our children our own fears and confusion regarding death. What happened between my mother and me at my grandfather's death is a good example. When we do this, we are giving our children faulty role models.

I think we should invite and bring all children to the visitation, from babes in arms to teenagers. They need preparation however, even the teenagers.

Generally a teen will say they don't want to attend the visitation. They want to remember "Grandpa as he was." A teen has one foot in childhood and one foot in adulthood, and by saying they would rather not attend they are really saying they are uncertain as to how to behave. Their concern is, will they do something that appears foolish. Our lack of appropriate role models is very evident in a teenager's response to visitations and funerals. Tell the teenager the very same things you would tell the four or five year old. Tell them what a visitation is, exactly what is going to happen, and what their role is during that time. Also give them an out by saying they can leave anytime they would like.

We don't want to force any child, of any age, to attend and participate in something they feel uncomfortable about, but generally with their fears neutralized through knowledge and understanding they will want to be part of the family gathering.

Although I encourage all children to attend the visitation, I do not think a funeral is a place for very small children, children from one to around five or six. A funeral is a ritual based on words. It is not interactive, but passive. We sit, we listen, and we seek comfort in words and song. If a child cannot understand the meaning of the words or the ritual or comprehend the reason for sitting quietly, then that child belongs somewhere else. A child talking, playing, or asking questions during the funeral service is distracting to everyone. The child is not receiving any benefit from the service, and neither is anyone else.

Each child is unique and their ability to grasp the seriousness of the moment is certainly individual, but if a child doesn't understand the solemness of church on Sunday, then they won't understand a funeral. It is best to leave them with a sitter. Let the church ladies watch them and then after the service get them for the ride to the cemetery and the gathering later.

Before the visitation, gather the children together to explain about the next few days. You can say that

Grandpa died, and when someone dies, we have a visitation. It is a gathering, with Grandpa's body, of our family and friends. It is a get together to visit and support each other. That's why we call it a visitation; we will be visiting. We will see Grandpa's body to say goodbye to it, and then we will be standing around talking. Sometimes we'll laugh because we may be remembering some of the funny things Grandpa did, and sometimes we'll be crying because we are sad that Grandpa won't be with us any more.

When someone dies, we put the body in a box called a coffin. It has fancy cloth inside and a pillow for Grandpa's head. Grandpa will be in his Sunday suit (or golf sweater, whatever is the family choice) and he will be lying in the box with his hands folded on his chest, with his eyes closed. And this is silly, but he will have his glasses on even though his eyes are closed.

Grandpa will have makeup on his face and even his hands. We can touch him but he won't feel like we do. He will feel cold and his skin won't move around like it used to. All this is what it is like to be dead.

There will be flowers around the coffin, and we are going to have pictures from our family albums on a table to look at and remember the good times we have had with Grandpa. This is our time to say goodbye to him. One of the ways we can say good-bye is to draw (or write a letter) to him. This is a way to show or say what is in our heart now that he is gone. It shows how sad we are and how much we are going to miss him. It is okay to cry because we are sad, and it is okay to laugh when we remember something funny. We will have all kinds of feelings.

The next day will probably be the funeral and again we tell the children about the service. It is like going to church on Sundays. If the child is small and not going to attend, explain "you get to play in the preschool at church just like on Sunday." After the service, there will be a ride in a special car and we will go to where Grandpa's body, in his coffin, is going to stay. Let the child run around and explore, with supervision, while the short interment service is conducted.

With these explanations, the child will have been included in the services, will have a simple understanding of the various emotions of grieving, and will have experienced death and its normal rituals. A responsible role model will have been established that can serve throughout the rest of life. Our first experience with death is our most memorable. It sets the foundation upon which we build our responses to future deaths.

LIVING WILL &
DURABLE POWER OF ATTORNEY

LIVING WILL

DURABLE POWER OF ATTORNEY

DO NOT RESUSITATE

NOTES:

In 1991, Congress passed a law called the Patient Self Determination Act.

The essence of this law was that patients have the right to make decisions regarding their care. This includes the right to accept or refuse medical or surgical treatment and the right to outline in advance the kind of care they want or don't want.

If we don't claim our right to make end of life decisions, then the medical profession will make them for us.

The medical model is disease-oriented. The goal is to treat the disease. Medical schools teach students to keep trying to fix and cure because what they learn from one success or failure may help another person somewhere, somehow. In the medical profession, death is generally seen as the enemy and a failure. When the emphasis is on disease, its treatment and cure instead of being on the people that have a disease, it is easy to see why death is looked at as a failure. The person becomes secondary.

Because of this disease orientation, in a living or death situation, most medical expertise is focused on fixing. That works very well most of the time. If I am in a car accident, I want everything possible done to fix me.

However, if I have a life threatening illness and my body can't be fixed, or the injuries from the car accident are not fixable, unless I have written instructions or someone to speak for me, most doctors will still do everything they can to fix me--even if I am not fixable. That is their job!

When we enter a hospital or a nursing facility, we are asked about our end of life wishes. If we can speak for ourselves--great, we get what we want.

However, if we are unable to communicate our wishes and have left no legal instructions, then it will be assumed we want everything possible done. That includes feeding tubes, ventilators, and heart resuscitation.

If we have definite ideas about our medical care, we need to have a Living Will and a Durable Medical Power of Attorney.

Most people are uncomfortable addressing end of life issues. Americans in particular have the idea if we talk about death and dying, then that means we will die. It infringes upon our illusion that we are going to live forever. Because our personal dying and death concept is so unreal, we procrastinate making decisions regarding our end of life experience.

I want to propose a change of perspective to the concept of dying. As I have mentioned previously, the word dying is a misnomer. We are either alive or we are dead. The space in between is called living. As long as we are breathing, we are living.

Operating from this perspective, then the question of advance directives (Living Will, Durable Medical Power of Attorneys and Do NOT Resuscitate) becomes not, "how I want to die?" but, "How I want to live until I am dead?"

A Living Will and a Durable Medical Power of Attorney are the closest we can come to insuring we be allowed to live to the end of our life the way we choose.

The best way to insure our end of life wishes are met is to tell our doctor and our family when we are sick, at the very moment the decisions have to be made, what we want done and not done. Ideally, we want to be an active participant in our treatment and our medical care. We want to be in control, making informed decisions. Unfortunately, we will probably not be in the position to express our wishes, and take charge of our destiny. We will probably be so incapacitated, even non-responsive, when decisions have to be made, that someone else will be making our end of living choices.

We need that person who speaks for us to be someone we trust implicitly. Someone who knows us, someone who understands what choices we would make. That person would have our Durable Medical Power of Attorney.

A Durable Medical Power of Attorney actually gives another person the legal power to make medical choices for us when we are unable to make them ourselves. It takes effect only when, due to whatever circumstances, we cannot make decisions for ourselves. A Durable Medical Power of Attorney is a legal document, but it does not have to be made out in the presence of an attorney. Two unrelated witnesses can sign the Durable Medical Power of Attorney form and it can be notarized. Simple, easy, just very thought-provoking and often very difficult to bring ourselves to do. It is only valid on medical issues, not financial ones. Financial would be a Power of Attorney.

We need to make sure that the person to whom we assign the Durable Medical Power of Attorney knows what we want concerning end of living issues. We need to talk to them in detail about our philosophy of life, living, medical choices and death. We need to specifically explain to them what we want and don't want in the area of treatment, hydration, feeding tubes, antibiotics, ventilators, and resuscitation. We need to fill out a Living Will and give it to the person to whom we have given our

Durable Medical Power of Attorney. Now they have our written instructions. Those written instructions will give the life and death decisions they will be making for us more credibility since they show our premeditated choices.

We should also carry a copy of our Living Will in an easily accessible place; inside a billfold is good, in case of an accident. Have with the Living Will the name and phone number of the person who has the Durable Medical Power of Attorney.

What is a Living Will? It is a written document that speaks for us when we can't speak for ourselves. It is a form we complete outlining the kind of medical care we want and don't want should we be in a life threatening situation and unable to participate in making a choice. It is not legally binding. It is only a written statement of medical intent

A Living Will is generally used at the doctor's discretion. That is why it is very important to discuss the Living Will with our primary physician so he/she knows first hand our thoughts on end of life issues and Advanced Directives.

Our family also needs to know our intentions, as well as the existence of the Living Will and who has our Durable Power of Attorney. None of this does any good if no one knows about it.

I have found in working with nursing facilities and even doctors and hospitals that if the family is not in agreement with a Living Will, the Living Will will not be honored. That is why a Durable Medical Power of Attorney is needed. That is why family discussion, as scary and difficult as it is, needs to happen.

I had a patient with a quiet, soft-spoken,

nonassertive husband. She had a Living Will but had not given anyone a Durable Medical Power of Attorney. When the patient became non-responsive in a nursing facility, the doctor transferred the patient to the hospital and put her on life support machines. When the husband reminded the doctor his wife had a Living Will, the doctor said he felt the patient had changed her mind about her Living Will and chose not honor it. The husband had no recourse but to see his wife die on life support machines.

It is also not good enough for the family to say, "Mom wants," or "Mom told me." Often a doctor will listen and act according to the family wishes, but if family members disagree amongst themselves as to what they want for Mom, then generally all medical options will be utilized.

In a nursing facility, generally, if even one family member disagrees as to whether a person should be placed on a No Code status, the facility will do a code. A code means that if you stop breathing for any reason the medical staff will do everything in their medical power to get you breathing again-- even if it is apparent to everyone involved that the attempt is futile. The fear of lawsuits often guides judgment and actions.

If one of our end of life choices is to not have anyone try to restart our heart should it stop, to not try to bring us back once we have died, then we need to have a signed Do Not Resuscitate (DNR) form. This form is only used if we have a life threatening illness, severe stroke that can't be fixed, irreversible coma or some situation where we have been deemed non-fixable and our heart has stopped or we have stopped breathing.

You would not want a DNR if you were fixable. You would not have one pre-signed with your Living

Will when you are healthy. It is only appropriate when you are facing the end of your life.

If you have a life threatening illness and die at home, once someone calls 911 and there is no Do Not Resuscitate form, the paramedics will do CPR, Cardio Pulmonary Resuscitation. They will try to restart the heart and your breathing. That is their job!

There is a specific DNR, Do Not Resuscitate, form. Generally that form can't be copied. It is gotten from hospitals, nursing homes, hospices or home health care agencies.

It is very difficult to address the issues presented in any of these forms. They force us to face our mortality. I asked my father, when he was in the last stages of lung cancer, to talk with me about his end of living wishes and about filling out a Do Not

Resuscitate form while he was in the hospital. His response was, "if I'm on life support machines for a week and the brain waves say I'm dead, for a week, then you can take me off the machines." We had a gentle talk, he signed a Do Not Resuscitate, and indeed died in the hospital.

My point in telling his story is that not everyone will want a Do Not Resuscitate. There is no right or wrong to this important decision. It is a matter of understanding what the alternatives are, of having someone honestly telling us our true choices. Then we can make an informed choice instead of an emotional choice.

Living Will, Durable Power of Attorney and Do Not Resuscitate options are available so that everyone can live their life challenges in the manner of their own choosing, not someone else's.

Health Care Treatment Directive

I,_____, make this Health Care Treatment Directive to
Print Name
exercise my right to determine the course of my health care and to provide clear and convinc-
ing proof of my treatment decisions **when I lack the capacity to make or communicate my
decisions** and there is no realistic hope that I will regain such capacity.

If my physician believes that a certain life prolonging procedure or other health care treatment
may provide me with comfort, relieve pain or lead to a significant recovery, I direct my physician to try the treatment for a reasonable period of time. However, if such treatment proves to
be ineffective, I direct treatment be withdrawn even if so doing may shorten my life.

I direct I be given health care treatment to relieve pain or to provide comfort even if such treatment might shorten my life, suppress my appetite or my breathing, or be habit-forming.

I direct all life prolonging procedures be withheld or withdrawn when there is no hope of
significant recovery, and I have:
 • a terminal condition; or
 • a condition, disease or injury without reasonable expectation that I will regain an
   acceptable quality of life; or
 • substantial brain damage or brain disease which cannot be significantly reversed.

1). When any of the above conditions exist, **I DO NOT WANT** the life prolonging
procedures which I have initialed below. (You should assume any treatments not
initialed may be administered to you.)
 • surgery .... _____ initials
 • heart-lung resuscitation (CPR).. _____ initials
 • antibiotics .... _____ initials
 • dialysis.. _____ initials
 • mechanical ventilator (respirator)... _____ initials
 • tube feedings (food and water delivered through a tube in the vein,
   nose or stomach)... _____ initials
 • other _____ .... _____ initials

2). I make other instructions as follows: **(You may describe what a minimally acceptable quality of life is for you.)**

_____

_____

_____

_____

If you do not wish to name an agent as referred to on the reverse side, initial here _____,
write "None" in the space provided for an agent's name, sign and have witnessed and/or notarized.

---

*Discuss this document and your ideas about quality of life with your agent, physician(s), family
members, friends and clergy and provide them with a signed copy (or photocopy thereof).* You may
evoke or change this document. Periodic review is recommended. If there are no changes after each
eview, initial and date in the margin.

This document is provided as a service by the Kansas City Metropolitan Bar Association and its founda-
on, the Metropolitan Medical Society of Greater Kansas City, Midwest Bioethics Center and the Missouri
Lawyer Trust Account Foundation.)

Durable Power of Attorney for Health Care Decisions

This is a Durable Power of Attorney for Heath Care Decisions, and the authority of my agent shall not terminate if I become incapacitated. I grant to my agent full authority to make decisions for me regarding my health care. In exercising this authority, my agent shall follow my desires as stated in my Health Care Treatment Directive or otherwise known to my agent. My agent's authority to interpret my desires is intended to be as broad as possible and any expenses incurred should be paid by my resources. My agent may not delegate the authority to make decisions. My agent is authorized as follows to:

> *If there is a statement in paragraphs 1 through 6 below with which you do not agree, draw a line through it and add your initials.*

1. Consent, refuse or withdraw consent to any care, treatment, service or procedure, (including artificially supplied nutrition and/or hydration/tube feeding) used to maintain, diagnose or treat a physical or mental condition;
2. Make decisions regarding organ donation, autopsy and the disposition of my body;
3. Make all necessary arrangements for any hospital, psychiatric hospital or psychiatric treatment facility, hospice, nursing home or similar institution; to employ or discharge health care personnel (any person who is licensed, certified or otherwise authorized or permitted by the laws of the state to administer health care) as the agent shall deem necessary for my physical, mental and emotional well being;
4. Request, receive and review any information, verbal or written, regarding my personal affairs or physical or mental health including medical and hospital records and to execute any releases of other documents that may be required in order to obtain such information;
5. Move me into or out of any state for t eh purpose of complying with my Health Care Treatment Directive or the decisions of my agent;
6. Take any legal action reasonably necessary to do what I have directed.

I appoint the following person to be my agent to make health care decisions for me WHEN AND ONLY WHEN I lack the capacity to make or communicate a choice regarding a particular health care decision and my Health Care Treatment Directive does not adequately cover circumstances. I request that the person serving as my agent be my guardian if one is needed.

> If you do not wish to name an agent, write "NONE" in the space provided below.

Agent's Name _____ Telephone: _____

Address: _____

If my agent is not available or not willing to make health care decisions for me or, if my agent is my spouse and is legally separated or divorced from me, I appoint the person or persons named below (in the order named if more than one listed) as my agent: **(It is not necessary to name an alternate agent.)**

First Alternate Agent	**Second Alternate Agent**
Name: _____	Name: _____
Address: _____	Address: _____
Telephone: _____	Telephone: _____

Protection of Persons Who May Rely on My Agent: I and my estate hold my agent and my caregivers harmless and protect them against any claim for following this durable power of attorney.
Severability: If any part of this document is held to be unenforceable under law, I direct that all of the other provisions of the document shall remain in force and effect.

Date: _____ **XSignature** _____

Witness _____ Date_____ Witness_____ Date _____

Notarization

> *Notarization of the Durable Power of Attorney is required in some states (e.g. Missouri but not Kansas). If this document is both witnessed and notarized, it is more likely to be honored in other states.*

On this _____ day of _____, 20 _____, before me personally appeared the aforesaid declarant, to me known to be the person described in and who executed the foregoing instrument and acknowledged that he/she executed the same as his/her free act and deed. IN WITNESS WHEREOF, I have hereunto set my hand and affixed my official seal in the County of _____, State of _____, the day and year first above written.

Notary Public: _____ Commission Expires: _____

Acceptance: (Optional) I have discussed this document with the person making this durable power of attorney and I accept the responsibility designated to me as stated above.

Date _____ Agent _____

FOR MORE INFORMATION CALL MIDWEST BIOETHICS CENTER • 816/756-1735

DO NOT RESUSCITATE
Prehospital DNR Request Form
An Advanced Request to Limit the Scope of Emergency Medical Care

I, _____ request the limited emergency care as herein described.

(Name)

I understand DNR means that if my heart stops beating or if I stop breathing, no medical procedure to restart breathing or heart functioning will be instituted.

I understand this decision will *not* prevent me from obtaining other emergency medical care by prehospital care providers or medical care directed by a physician prior to my death.

I understand I may revoke this directive at any time.

I give permission for this information to be given to the prehospital care providers, doctors, nurses, or other health care personnel as necessary to implement this directive.

I hereby agree to the "Do Not Resuscitate" (DNR) directive.

_____   _____
Signature   Date

Witness:*

Witness:_____ Date: _____

Address _____

*Must be 18 or older, not related to the declarant by blood or marriage, not entitled to any portion of the declarant's estate according to Kansas laws of intestate succession or under any will of the declarant or codicil thereto, and not directly financially responsible for the declarant's medical care expenses.

Attending physician:* I AFFIRM THIS DIRECTIVE IS THE EXPRESSED WISH OF THE PATIENT, IS MEDICALLY APPROPRIATE, AND IS DOCUMENTED IN THE PATIENT'S PERMANENT MEDICAL RECORD.
In the event of an acute cardiac or respiratory arrest, no cardiopulmonary resuscitation will be initiated.

_____   _____
Attending Physician's Signature*   Date

_____   _____
Address   Facility or Agency Name

*Signature of physician is not required if the above-named is a member of a church or religion which, in lieu of medical care and treatment, provides treatment by spiritual means through prayer alone and care consistent therewith in accordance with the tenets and practices of such church or religion.

Revocation Provision
I hereby revoke the above declaration.

_____   _____
Signature   Date

EPILOGUE

WHAT MY HEART, MIND & SOUL
HAS LEARNED

FROM MY HEART

WITH MY MIND

IN MY SOUL

NOTES:

This is the point where I share with you what I have learned from areas deep within about living in and leaving this world. I debated a long time about whether to include my perspectives on life. Would it be considered too philosophical, maybe even preachy? Would it be considered presumptuous of me to share my personal thoughts? After much internal deliberation, I decided to risk showing some of what is under my social mask in the hopes it will give others further insights.

If I had not gotten into Hospice work, I probably would never have developed the insights I want to share. Working with people on end of life issues has been a wake up call for me to life. It has shown me just how precious and precarious the days, weeks, months and years are. It taught me that we need to grab the ring or it will pass us by and be gone forever.

Oprah has a feature in her magazine called, "What I Know for Sure." The following is what I know for sure today, tomorrow might revise my thoughts and cause me to think differently. Change is life. There isn't one without the other.

FROM MY HEART

I have learned that most of us provide love with expectations and conditions. Our love is based on our history, our culture, and our beliefs. Unconditional love is a rarity. It is rare because it is so difficult to give.

It is a lot easier to unconditionally care for a stranger than to accept our own family. A stranger brings no baggage, no past to the relationship. We have the opportunity to see the person in the now, as simply whom they present at the moment. Of course we have to put aside our stereotypes, our preconceived ideas about the person before we can truly be in the present with them.

Dr. Elizabeth Kuebler-Ross uses the metaphor of a coffee pot. Explaining how you pour clear water through the coffee grounds and the resulting coffee is "colored water." Personalities are "poured through" our brains, resulting in a tainted picture of the person--tainted by our belief systems, culture, fears, environment, childhood, judgments, expectations, and insecurities. All those things that make us who we are affect how we perceive others. Given all this, it is still easier to be open with a stranger who has not touched us in our heart, who has not caused us to hurt.

Over the years, most of the people I have taken care of I have cared for as children of God. Physically I cared for them with the respect and dignity that a human being is entitled too. Every so often, however, a person would creep into my heart and Barbara would become involved. Those people filled an empty space within me.

When I started in hospice, I made a deal with myself that there would be people who touched my heart in a personal way and that I would grieve for them when they were gone. Rather than miss the relationship, I agreed to feel those losses.

I can recall the names and faces of those special people, the father I wished I had, the best friend, the peer, the children. If all of my patients and their families got into my heart the way those people did, I would not have been able to continue, my heart would have grieved too much. It would have also been necessary to consider why my heart and life were so empty that I was using my patients to fill them.

I learned to be grateful for all the blessings life has

given me, for the air I breathe in so easily, for the warmth of feeling the sun on my skin without pain, for the food I eat with gusto and in abundance, for the feet and legs that carry me gracefully and freely on my daily walks. I am grateful for my wonderful life and the caring people in it. I appreciate life since I know how short and unpredictable this adventure can be.

This life is for doing. The only opportunity for experiencing is when I am in my physical body. I can ruminate when I am dead. My mantra has become, "If not now, when?"

WITH MY MIND

Appreciating the brevity of life, I see that regrets are a waste. I am a timid soul who approaches life cautiously and sometimes with reticence, so that each night I ask myself, "For what have I traded a day of my life? Are there any regrets about today, and can

I amend them?" If I don't wake up in the morning, I want to make sure that I will have no unfinished business to haunt me or those I care about.

Our attitude toward life affects its grandeur. Using the old cliché, I can view my place in this world as a cup half full or half empty. I can look through eyes that search for fault or look for good. What I look for, I will find.

I have heard many cries of anguish that say, "Why me?" My mind's response is always, "Why not you?" Difficult events happen in life for all of us; that is what life is about--reacting to the situations that are presented to us. Life is hard work. It is choices. It is attitude. It is not what happens to us throughout our sojourn into living, but how we deal with those happenings.

Most of us go through life on automatic pilot. We

are not really aware of the living we are doing. We don't question why we think and react the way we do, we just react. We perform our routines; we interact with others just as we always have day after day after day. We proceed through life like little gerbils running on a wheel. We keep moving but go nowhere. Get up in the morning, drink our coffee, get ready for work, get the kids off to school, drive to work, do our job, come home, fix dinner, watch a little television (more than likely do laundry, tidy the house) get the kids ready for bed and crash into bed ourselves. The next morning we begin all over again. Around and around we go, one foot in front of the other, again and again and again.

I don't think most of us are thinking, and perceiving. In our rush we miss the full moon, the rustle of the leaves, and sometimes even the voices of others.

Everything we do in our life, we do out of our own

needs, for ourselves. The idea that we are helping others is a misnomer. We are first and foremost helping ourselves; if others are helped in the process, that is a side effect, not a primary effect. Even the acts we perform that harm us, that make us uncomfortable, are done from past habits, memories and behaviors. Those acts make us feel a sort of comfort in their uncomfortableness.

When I was in nursing school, a teacher asked us to write an essay on, "Why I want to be a nurse?" She qualified the assignment by saying, "And I don't want you to say it's because you want to help people," which is exactly why I thought I was getting into nursing. By looking deeper, I learned I wanted to be a nurse because my mother wanted me to be a nurse and I was a people pleaser, particularly a mother pleaser. Unfortunately, I didn't learn this about myself for another twenty-five years. I don't even remember what answer I gave the teacher.

If we can examine the emotional wounds and scars, childhood patterning, spiritual indoctrination, mental conditioning and beliefs we've accumulated over the years, we have the opportunity to refine and/or eliminate that which is no longer necessary for functional, alert living. Without a lot of old conditioning, and with a conscious effort to know ourselves, to be aware of our world and actions in it, we can start taking charge of our lives instead of letting life happen to us.

I have learned that I want to live a purposeful and directed life. A life that, through the aware choices I make, I can find fulfillment.

An important part of this life experience is our interaction with others. There certainly is no perfect relationship. Relationships are evolving, growing and changing all the time as the people in them change. Sometimes we grow together and sometimes we grow apart. This isn't good and it isn't bad. It just happens.

Because of the uncertainty of living, I think we need to do and say daily what is on our minds and in our hearts. Resolve the hurts with others even if we have to be the one to make the first effort for reconciliation. We need to let people know often that we care about them, say the thank yous and the I love yous frequently, and let go of our personal expectations for other's behavior.

A big part of what patients and families have taught me is about time and what we do with it. There is really only this moment, now. What I do in this moment is of great import. What I have done in the past is only a memory, actually a distorted memory because it has come through my "coffee pot," The future is only my imagination, what I hope to create. Now, right this moment, is real, the only real we have. How many of us appreciate and consciously participate in each given piece of time?

IN MY SOUL

Working with death on a daily basis for years actually forced me to look for reasons for being alive. It made me ask the question, "What is the purpose of living?"

From a lot of searching and questioning, I have come to accept that life is a Divine Opportunity to experience; that every occurrence, easy or difficult, is an ordained occasion; and in the midst of these experiences, we are to achieve peace of mind, joy and fulfillment. Put more simply, everything happens for a reason and in spite of all that is happening, our life's job is to find peace of mind, joy and fulfillment.

Bringing peace of mind, joy and fulfillment to each experience that life offers is a big challenge. It seems like it is a lot easier to do things that are self-destructive than to do constructive living. Eating healthy, exercising, thinking positive thoughts are hurdles we face daily. It is so easy to get caught up in each day's activities as we ride our "gerbil wheel," that we forget to look for joy. We lose whatever peace of mind we might have and our sense of fulfillment is lost in our need to just get through another day.

In his book Conversations With God, Neale Donald Walsch says, "I (God) have sent you nothing but angels." What a profound statement! It can be interpreted in so many ways. After thinking a lot about what "I have sent you nothing but angels" means, I finally settled on a message of reassurance. Reassurance that every occurrence in our life is a Divine Gift. Every person, every place, every situation, whether it is perceived as positive or negative, is a Divine Opportunity, an angel.

If I can live my life from the perspective that all is as it should be, that all is an opportunity for me to experience, that every person and event is a Divine Occurrence, then fear and uncertainty gives way to peace of mind--most of the time. We are all still works in progress.

Watching birds feeding at the feeder, listening to the rain in the trees, reading a good book in a shady outdoor spot, most of nature brings me joy. Also there is joy in sharing dreams and ideas with a special friend, just being silly, or finding and experiencing real laughter.

Being creative, doing for others (voluntarily, not out of obligation), and doing a task fully and with pride can give a sense of fulfillment.

Fulfillment affects our sense of self worth. We feel "full," more complete, as a result of an activity or interaction. I wonder if some of us don't look for fulfillment in empty places by basing our worth on employment, status, possessions and money.

And finally, I've learned that as we are born so we must die. Nothing is permanent, nothing is forever. Time consistently moves us in the direction of death and yet it is in that very time, each moment, that life is felt and experienced. Each second gives us the opportunity to be, to do, to see, to hear, to feel-- while that same second takes us closer to the final act of living.

INTERESTING READING

The Good Death; Webb, Marilyn; Bantam Books; 1997

Learning to Die; Mundy, John; Spiritual Frontiers Fellowship, 1977

Philosophy of Death And Dying; Kamath, M.V.; Himalayan International Institute of Science and Philosophy, 1978

The Transition Called Death; Hampton, Charles; Theosophical Publishing; 1979

Who Dies? Levine, Stephen; Anchor Press/ Doubleday; 1982

Midwives to the Dying; Schmeider RN BSN, Miriam; Selliken Bernard RN BSN, Jan; Angel's Work Publishing; 1992

The Tibetan Book of Living & Dying; Rinpoche, Sogyal; Harper Collins, 1992

To Die Well; Reoch, Richard; Harper Perennial; 1996

Hard Choices for Loving People; Dunn, Hank; A&A Publishers Inc; 1994

Death, The Final Stage of Growth; Kubler-Ross, Elizabeth; Touchstone Books; 1975

Questions & Answers on Death & Dying; Kubler-Ross, Elizabeth; Touchstone Books; 1997

Death: The Great Adventure; Bailey, Alice; Lucis Publishing Company; 1985

Helping a Child Understand Death; Vogel, Linda Jane; Fortress Press; 1975

Final Gifts; Callanan, Maggie & Kelley, Patricia; Bantam Books; 1992

Life At Death; Ring, Kenneth; PH.D.; Coward, McCann and Geoghegan; 1980

Life After Life; Moody, Raymond; Mockingbird Books; 1975

Love is the Link; Kercher, Pamela, MD 1995

On Life After Death; Kubler-Ross, Elizabeth; Celestial Arts; 1991

The Seven Spiritual Laws of Success; Chopra, Deepak; Amber-Allen Publishing; 1993

No Ordinary Moments; Millman, Dan; H.J. Kramer, Inc; 1992

The Fountain Of Age; Friedan, Betty; Simon & Schuster; 1993

The Thief of the Spirit; Hammerschlag, M.D., Carl; RGA Publishing Group; 1992

Why People Don't Heal And How They Can; Myss, Caroline PhD; Random House; 1997

Anatomy of the Spirit; Myss, Caroline PhD; Random House; 1996

New Passages; Sheely, Gail; Random House; 1995

Conversations With God, Book I; Walsch, Neale Donald; G.P. Putnam's Sons; 1996

Conversations With God, Book II; Walsch, Neale Donald; Hampton Roads; 1997

Conversations With God, Book III; Walsch, Neale Donald; Hampton Roads; 1998

The 10 Greatest Gifts I Give My Children; Vannoy, Steven W.; Simon & Schuster; 1994

Parent Effectiveness Training; Gordon, Dr. Thomas; New American Library; 1970

I'm Here To Help; Ray Catherine M; Hospice Handouts, a division of MCRay

Company; 1992

I Don't Know What To Say; Buckman, Dr. Robert; Vintage Books; 1988

Beyond Grief; Staudacher, Carol; New Hardings Publications;

Grief Counseling & Grief Therapy; Worden PhD, William J; Springer Publishing; 1982

How Many Times Can You Say Goodbye?; Pardoe, Jenifer; The Liturgical Press;1991

Remember The Secret; Kubler-Ross, Elizabeth; Celestial Arts; 1982

Surviving, Healing & Growing, The Workbook; McWilliams, Peter; Prelude Press; 1991

How To Survive The Loss of a Love; McWilliams, Peter; Prelude Press; 1991

Symptom Control in Hospice & Palliative Care; Kaye, Peter; Hospice Education Institute; 1988

The Dehydration Question; Nursing; January 1983

The American Way of Dying; US News & World Report; December. 4, 1995

Terminal Dyspnea: A Hospice Approach; Horn, Lori W. American Journal of Hospice & Palliative Care; March/April. 1992

Nutrition & Hydration in Hospice Care; Gallagher-Alred, C; O'Rawe Amenta, M; The Haworth Press; 1993

Artificial Nutrition & Hydration of the Dying Patient; Ascheman, Pat, RN, OCN; Home Care Highlights, March 1996

Terminal Dehydration: A Review; Meares, Candace Jans, RN MSN; The American Journal of Hospice & Palliative Care; May/June 1994

Patient-Induced Dehydration-Can It Ever Be Therapeutic?; Smith, Shirley Ann RN MSN, OCN; Oncology Nursing Forum, Vol. 22 November 1995

Palliative Medicine; Woodruff, Roger; Asperula Pty Ltd Melbourne; 1996

Primer of Palliative Care; Storey, Peter MD; American Acad. of Hospice & Palliative Medicine; 1996

American Journal of Hospice Care: Healing the Dying Person; Karnes, Barbara; Gyulay, Jody; Fall, 1984

American Journal of Hospice Care: The Spiritual Moment of Death; Karnes, Barbara; September/October 1987

Gone From My Sight, the dying experience; Booklet; Karnes, Barbara; 1987

My Friend, I Care, the grief experience; Booklet; Karnes, Barbara; 1991

A Time To Live, living with a life threatening illness; Booklet; Karnes, Barbara; 1994

American Journal of Hospice Care; An Expressed Concern; Karnes, Barbara; March/April 1997

I realize the publishing dates on some of these resources and recommended reading date back to 1975. I have included them because I believe some of the information contained in these materials is timeless. The dynamics of dying do not necessarily change with time. Fluid still fills the lungs in an over hydrated dying person, the kidneys still shut down. Our advances in medicine cannot affect the natural dying process. Grief is grief, and its process is also unchanging.

In addition, this entire book is only my perceptions, my ideas, how Barbara Karnes views dying. These books helped form those perceptions. It took twenty-eight years of reading, studying, experiencing and building to reach today.

OTHER PUBLICATIONS

BY

BARBARA KARNES

Gone From My Sight, the dying experience

The biggest fear of watching someone die is fear of the unknown; not knowing what dying will be like or when death will actually occur.

This 14 page, large print booklet explains in a simple, gentle, yet direct manner the process of dying from disease.

Dying from disease is not like it is portrayed in the movies. Yet movies, not life, have become our role model. Death from disease is not happenstance. It doesn't just occur; there is a process. People die in stages of months, weeks, days and hours.

"Gone From My Sight" helps people understand dying, their own or someone else.

My Friend, I Care, the grief experience

Grief is as foreign to us as death. The experience is forced upon us by life situations that have been beyond our control. We become angry, depressed, fearful, and anxious. We do not know that all these feelings together represent grief: a normal, natural response to the loss of someone or something.

This 14 page, large print booklet is intended for the newly grieving. It addresses the normalness of grieving while offering suggestions for moving forward into living. It can be used as a sympathy card as it offers an expression of caring at the some time giving support and guidance.

Like its companions, "Gone From My Sight" and "A Time To Live," this booklet is written in a simple, direct, yet gentle manner.

A Time To Live, living with a life threatening illness

When a person receives the diagnosis of a life threatening illness, life as they know it ceases; never to return. They find themselves in uncharted territory having no guidelines to follow. Often they go home, sit down in their favorite recliner and stop living. All activity becomes centered around the disease and treatment. Fear and uncertainty replaces confidence and self- identity.

This 13 page, large print booklet is appropriate for anyone who is faced with the unpredictability of their future due to a life threatening illness. It offers guidance for living! It addresses issues everyone would do well to ponder and then goes a step further to explain comfort control, nutrition and sleep as it relates to serious illness.

RESOURCES

National Hospice and Palliative Care Organization
1700 Diagonal Road, Suite 625
Alexandria, VA 22314
(703) 837-1500 • Fax (703) 837-1233
Toll free (800) 646-6460
Web site: www.nhpco.org

National Association for Home Care and Hospice
228 Seventh Street, SE
Washington, DC 20003
(202) 547-7424 • Fax (202) 547-3540
Web site: www.nahc.org

Compassionate Friends: grief support after the death of a child
(630) 990-0010 • Toll free (877) 969-0010
Web site: www.compassionatefriends.org

**COMFORT, SUPPORTIVE, PALLIATIVE CARE, HOSPICE or
HOME HEALTH:** look in the yellow pages under hospice and home
health

RECIPE FOR PROTEIN SUPPLEMENT
1 package instant breakfast
8 ounces of whole or soy milk
2 scoops of any flavored ice cream (or as many as you would like for
desired thickness)
1 TBS malt, fruit, chocolate, peanut butter or whatever else is pleasing
　　Combine ingredients in a blender. Serve in a small glass. Refrigerate
or freeze the remainder to use every 2 hours
　　Instant breakfast can be purchased in grocery stores in the breakfast
and cereal aisles
　　Ready-made protein supplements can be purchased in pharmacies,
discount stores and some grocery stores.

SOURCES OF PROTEIN are soy products, eggs, chicken, turkey,
fish, dairy products (custards, pudding, ice cream, cheese, cottage
cheese, milk and whey).

ABOUT THE AUTHOR

Barbara Karnes is a registered nurse. She began in Hospice as a volunteer in 1981, and since then has been a staff nurse, Clinical Director, Patient Care Manager and an Executive Director, all in the Hospice arena. She was the Director of the Hospice and Home Health Agencies for Olathe Medical Center in Olathe, KS, a suburb of Kansas City from 1989 until May of 1994. Since 1994 she has been presenting workshops and lectures throughout the country.

Barbara is the author of the booklets "Gone From My Sight", "My Friend, I Care," and "A Time To Live."

ORDER FORM

<u>The Final Act of Living:</u>   QTY
Reflections of a Long Time Hospice Nurse . . . . $15.00_____
shipping and handling included

<u>Gone From My Sight:</u>   QTY
The Dying Experience. . . . . $2.00_____
Available in Spanish, French, Russian & Italian

<u>My Friend, I Care:</u>   QTY
The Grief Experience . . . . $2.00_____
Available in Spanish

<u>A Time to Live:</u>   QTY
Living with a Life-Threatening Illness . . . . $2.00_____
Available in Spanish

Total # of Copies_____
Amount Paid _____

Shipping & Handling for $2.00 booklets:

1-2 . . . .$1.00	5-10 . . . . . .$3.00	26-50 . . . . .$5.00
3-4 . . . .$2.00	11-25 . . . . .$4.00	51-100 . . . .$7.00

Name _____

Address_____

City _____ State ___Zip _____

Phone _____

MAIL TO:
BARBARA KARNES BOOKS
PO BOX 189
DEPOE BAY, OR 97341